AROM

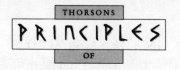

THORSONS
PRINCIPLES
OF

AROMATHERAPY

CATHY HOPKINS

Thorsons
An Imprint of HarperCollinsPublishers

Thorsons
An Imprint of HarperCollins*Publishers*
77–85 Fulham Palace Road
Hammersmith, London W6 8JB
1160 Battery Street
San Francisco, California 94111–1213
Published by Thorsons 1996

1 3 5 7 9 10 8 6 4 2

A catalogue record for this book
is available from the British Library

ISBN 0 7225 3263 6

Printed in Great Britain by
HarperCollinsManufacturing Glasgow

The publishers would like to thank
Jillie Collings for her suggestion for
the title of this series *Principles of . . .*

CONTENTS

INTRODUCTION

I n the first half of this century, aromatherapy was still relatively unknown to the general public. Today, almost every woman's magazine you pick up recommends it, either for its healing and therapeutic properties or simply for the sheer pleasure and relaxation of the experience. And yet, it is not a treatment exclusive to women. Over the last decade, an increasing number of men have also discovered it, amongst other things, as a valuable aid for combating the ever-increasing enemy of all of us in this day and age – stress.

There's no doubt that aromatherapy is the most enjoyable and luxurious of all the alternative treatments but it should not be overlooked for its potency as a therapy. Each of the oils contains healing properties, for example all the oils are natural antiseptics, others are antibiotic, others antiviral and so on. The correct usage of the oils can improve a whole variety of ailments from those common to all of us (flu, headaches, stress) to the more individual complaints (cellulite, bad circulation, palpitations).

The aim of this book is to introduce the principles of this fascinating therapy. Then, with a comprehensive knowledge of the fundamentals of the essential oils and their application, the reader will be able to gain maximum usage and benefit from them in everyday life.

WHAT IS AROMATHERAPY?

A romatherapy is the use of aromatic essential oils for both physical and psychological benefit. Despite enormous media coverage from TV, magazines and books, it is still a mystery to many. 'Isn't that something to do with scented oils?' I'm often asked when I mention the subject. Others know that there are different oils for different conditions but have no idea how they are used.

This chapter will briefly explain what aromatherapy is, some aspects of which I will elaborate upon more in later chapters.

WHAT AROMATHERAPY IS:

- The use of essential oils for health and relaxation as well as being the most pleasurable and luxurious of the alternative treatments.

- The only treatment that combines remedies with hands on therapy and body work.

- It is most effective when used as a preventative therapy rather than curative.

- It is a holistic treatment, that is: one that takes into account the whole body and lifestyle of a person and aims to treat the root of the problem and not just the symptom.

- A therapy that treats the mind and emotions as well as the physical body.

Aroma means scent or fragrance, therapy means treatment, therefore aromatherapy literally translated means a treatment that has a therapeutic effect as a result of this scent. This, although true, is the cause of what is perhaps the biggest misunderstanding of all about the oils. For, aromatherapy is much more than simply subjecting a client to a series of different smells. Perhaps it is because of the word 'aroma' therapy that some people think that the healing claims about the oils only relate to the scent. In fact, some practitioners prefer to call the oils 'essential' oils rather than 'aromatherapy' oils as it is the plant essence that is used in the treatment rather than just the scent. Although each oil does have its own unique and individual smell, some flowery and pleasant (ylang-ylang, lavender), some menthol (eucalyptus, peppermint), some woody (sandalwood, benzoin), and others sharp and refreshing (lime, grapefruit), this aroma and its effect on the limbic part of our brain is only a part of the therapeutic power of the oils.

The oils are made up of components which have healing properties. Once these have entered the system (through the skin with massage or the lungs in inhalation) they can get on with their healing work and improve a whole variety of conditions.

WHAT THE ESSENTIAL OILS ARE:

The oils are aromatic, volatile substances which have been extracted from various natural sources such as fruits, plants, herbs, tree barks and roots. All the plant sources used for aromatherapy are known to have beneficial healing properties.

Although these essences have been used in medicine and perfumes for thousands of years it is only in the last 20 years that they have really come to the attention of the British media and general public. The result of this is that the oils are now on sale in most health shops around the country. Despite there being some 400 oils actually known in the world, there are only approximately 80 oils available. Of those 80, some are used much more frequently (for example, lavender) while others are hardly used at all (for example, hyssop). Most aromatherapists will keep around 30–40 for their practice and most home users can get by quite sufficiently with a neat dozen. They come in small, dark glass bottles containing 5, 10 or 20 mg of oil and are sold in their concentrate form. The price can vary quite considerably depending on availability and quality. For example, lavender oil is usually easy to obtain and can cost around £3.00 for 10 ml whereas only 5 ml of rose oil can cost between £25-£40. Don't let this put you off! Most of the oils are well within the budget of most households and in Chapter 5 I'll recommend which oils are the best buy for common usage.

Precaution

As some of the oils are toxic, and others can burn if used in excess, most of the oils should be diluted before use, particularly if they are to be applied directly to the skin. It is important for anyone interested in using the oils at home to study the precautions and directions for home use (see Chapter 3). Once these few rules have been firmly grasped, home use can be safe, easy and beneficial.

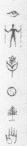

PROPERTIES OF THE OILS

Analgesic, antibiotic, antifungal, antiseptic, antiviral, aphrodisiac, diuretic, expectorant, laxative, sedative, tonic, stimulant to name but a few (see Appendices for a complete index).

Most of the oils combine some of these properties. Natural doesn't mean ineffective, for example tea tree oil is antiseptic, antibiotic, antifungal, and antiviral. It is four times stronger than most household disinfectants and yet it is still kind to the skin.

HANDS ON THERAPY

Hands on work is where the practitioner touches the client. Osteopathy, acupuncture, any kind of massage are all categorized as hands on therapy. This is opposed to the treatment when you are given a remedy to take but no physical contact between practitioner and client takes place. Aromatherapy combines both hands on and remedies through massage – one of the most effective ways of applying the essential oils. During the massage, the oils, which are diluted down into a base oil such as grapeseed or almond oil, are absorbed through the skin and into the bloodstream where they can start to do their work.

OTHER METHODS OF APPLYING THE OILS (SEE ALSO CHAPTER 3)

- Inhalation: particularly good for chest, nasal and throat infections.

- Compress: hot or cold, e.g. a hot compress with oil of camomile for period pains can be very soothing. A cold compress with peppermint on the forehead for a headache or with camomile on a swelling sprain can be very relieving.

- Vaporization: burning the oils, e.g. eucalyptus is one I always recommend to be burnt in offices, particularly in that run up to Christmas when everyone goes down with flu and colds. Amongst other things, eucalyptus is antiviral and can kill a virus and germs in the air.

- Baths: an aromatic bath is perhaps the simplest of all methods. Adding 6–8 drops of essential oil enhances any bathtime and not just because of the scent. Oil of lavender could be used after a long stressful day to aid relaxation, oil of bergamot could be used in the morning to get a weary, sluggish system fit for a new day.

AROMATHERAPY AS A HOLISTIC TREATMENT

A holistic treatment means that the practitioner will take into account a person's whole lifestyle and all their various complaints before prescribing treatment (in the aromatherapist's case, choosing particular oils for that individual). They do this in an effort to discover and treat the root of the condition rather than just the symptoms in which case the condition reappears.

As each person is unique, taking into account the individual symptoms helps assess which is going to be the most effective combination of oils. For example, someone may be complaining of stress. The stress may be physical, in which case a massage of the shoulders, lower back and neck with lavender to unwind would be beneficial. However, it may be that the person's stress is mainly inward, perhaps they haven't been sleeping well in which case one of the oils good for deep anxiety such as melissa or marjoram to promote a good night's rest would be best, together with a general massage giving particular attention to the feet to help promote a feeling of well-being (reflexology is often combined with aromatherapy and can help aid relaxation).

CONDITIONS THAT BENEFIT FROM AROMATHERAPY (SEE ALSO CHAPTER 13)

The benefits of aromatherapy are many and varied. With very few exceptions, everyone can gain from essential oils, no matter how mild or serious their condition . They can invigorate or relax. They can help sleep, relieve stress, constipation, swelling, backache, cellulite, heartburn, prevent premature ageing and they can be used at different stages in pregnancy to relieve symptoms and aid labour. Some oils are diuretic and some aphrodisiac.

THE OILS AS A PREVENTATIVE

There is no doubt that the most effective usage of the oils is as a preventative measure. I can speak from personal experience with this as many years ago I suffered from bronchitis which left me with a weakness in the chest. Knowing how debilitating this condition can be, I used to dread winter when everyone starts coughing and wheezing as I was always one of the first to fall ill. Now if I feel the slightest congestion in my lungs or if I'm in contact with anyone with a chest complaint, out comes the steam inhaler and the oils of pine and eucalyptus. I regularly inhale each day until I feel a hundred per cent again and for the past eight years I have never suffered more than a minor cough. I put this down to regular use of the appropriate oils as a preventative measure.

One of the truly remarkable things about essential oils is their ability to enhance mood and lift depression as well as benefit a person physically. Certain oils, apart from the pleasure of their scent, can raise low spirits or revive a flagging mind. For example, basil is particularly good for times when the brain feels overloaded and concentration is wavering. A few drops of basil oil on a tissue brought out and inhaled mid-afternoon in a stuffy office can wake up and recharge the most weary brain.

Jasmine, ylang-ylang and rose on the other hand are all oils which in their own individual ways can lift depression, jasmine being known to evoke joy, rose to heal and soothe, ylang-ylang to mellow.

In ancient Egyptian times, essential oils were a part of the armies' war plans. Invigorating oils such as bergamot or rosemary would be used to stimulate before going into battle, soothing oils such as lavender or camomile used to calm and unwind on return.

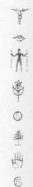

A HISTORICAL PERSPECTIVE

Although aromatherapy has only become popular in the last 10 to 15 years, it is actually an age old treatment dating back to the ancient civilizations of Egypt, China, Arabia, India, Greece and Rome.

Since that time, there have been references to it in the art, literature and medical journals of many different cultures. The history of the oils and their use make a colourful and fascinating story. Their popularity has rollercoasted up and down throughout the ages; now once again people seem to be rediscovering the benefits of what many of our ancient ancestors knew to be nature's healing gift.

EGYPT

The ancient Egyptians are generally regarded to be the founders of aromatherapy and were using aromatics as far back as 4,500 BC. Cleopatra (68–30 BC) was said to have applied her knowledge of the oils when seducing Anthony, selecting the oils of jasmine and rose, both of which are noted for their aphrodisiac properties.

Traces of the oils have been discovered in the tombs of ancient Egyptians. For example, when in 1897, the tomb of ruler King Menes who founded the city of Memphis in 3,000 BC was opened, it contained the remnants of aromatic products. In 1922, vases and ointments containing frankincense and spikenard were found in the tomb of Tutankhamun which dates back to 1,320 BC. It is said that even after all this time the fragrance of the oils was still discernible.

There are two explanations as to why oils would have been found in the tombs and pyramids. Firstly, the ancient Egyptians believed in the afterlife. They thought they could take their worldly goods with them. Hence many of the tombs were full of treasures and riches, all buried with the owner so that when he woke up in the afterlife, his riches would be there waiting for him. As the aromatic oils were considered very precious for health and beauty, they would have been part of the wealth stashed alongside the mummy.

Secondly, the oils were used for embalming. Traces of the oil of spikenard, cedarwood, cypress, frankincense, myrrh, nutmeg, clove and cinnamon have been found impregnated in mummies' bandages. These oils would have been used for their antiseptic and antibacterial properties to help preserve the bodies. In the case of the royals, they thought that the embalming protection of the oils would help them to arrive in the other world of the afterlife intact. In fact, the embalming was remarkably effective as fragments of intestine examined under microscope were found to be in remarkable condition even after thousands of years. Sadly, it seems that these oils were only available for use by royalty and the richer classes while others less fortunate were all dumped in a communal pit.

The ancient Egyptians also used the oils for cosmetics, beauty, massage and healing purposes. If you ever have the chance to visit Egypt you will see on many of the walls of the temples that there are beautiful hieroglyphics showing the people either offering scents to each other or receiving treatments from bowls or vases full of flower and plant substances. Egyptian ladies would have aromatic baths after which they would be massaged by slaves using aromatic ointments and oils.

These unguents weren't only made up for their scent but also to protect the skin, for example the eye make-up they wore would also protect the eyes from infection because of the healing components of the oils.

Egyptian perfume had the reputation that French has today as the place that truly knew how to create memorable scent. The temple at Edfou has a room containing inscriptions detailing formulas for many different types of perfume, some made up to stimulate and refresh, others concocted to sedate and evoke a meditative state. One of the best known perfumes from that time was Kyphi, said to have been made up from 16 different essences. Calamus, myrrh, juniper, mastic, cinnamon, cassia, spikenard, cyperus, henna, terebinth, frankincense and saffron are said to have been some of what surely must be the world's first perfume, the Chanel No 5 of ancient times.

Although today's perfumes may smell delightful, they don't have the healing or mind-expanding potential that ancient Kyphi must have had according to what Plutarch later wrote about the scent.

> The smell of this perfume penetrates your body through the nose. It makes you feel well and relaxed, the mind floats and you may find yourself in a dreamy state of happiness as if listening to beautiful music.

Frankincense, one of the rumoured components of Kyphi, is known to expand consciousness and spiritually uplift. Perhaps this is why even today it is still burnt in some churches. As well as for their fragrance, the oils were used by the Egyptians for their antiseptic, antiviral, antibacterial properties. They would have protected any wearer from disease and any infections in the air.

In the Papyrus Ebers, dated as far back as 1,550 BC, recipes and remedies were found for various ailments. The scrolls show physicians, priests and surgeons recommending inhalations, compresses and gargles. The priests would use the oils for the relief of various illnesses, making potions, pills and unguents. Mostly the ointments that have been found have shown that the oils were obtained by means of infusion. This involves leaving the plant material in a base oil of fat in the sun. After a few days, the base fat would have been permeated with the aroma – which can still be detected today, after 3,000 years.

Still other hieroglyphics show the ancients burning oils. Many of the doctors were also priests and they would dedicate oils to different gods, myrrh to the moon god, frankincense to Ra the sun god, artemisia to Isis, marjoram to Osiris.

CHINA

It seems that at the same time that the Egyptians were using aromatics, the ancient Chinese were also aware of their benefits.

In 2,000 BC, Kiwang-Ti, emperor of China, wrote a book detailing his discoveries regarding the properties of certain plants. In 2,650 BC the *Yellow Emperor's Classic of Internal Medicine* contained references to essential oils. The Great Herbal dated around 2,700 BC and named after Shen Nong listed 365 plants used medicinally. Close to the 400 oils that we have listed today.

In *Pen Ts'ao on Materia Medica of Li Shih Chen*, dated approximately 1529, 23 of the oils are described.

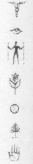

Essence of rose: this was for the liver, stomach and also an anti-depressant.

Jasmine: a general tonic for all organs of the body.

Camomile: for dizziness, headaches, colds.

Ginger: malaria, mucousy coughs.

Such references in these texts demonstrate that what many call a new age therapy is in fact one of the oldest therapies known to man.

INDIA

As with Egypt and China, it is commonly thought that the Indian culture has always known about the healing power of aromatics. There was a container found in the foothills of the Himalayas dating as far back as 3,000 BC. Evidence suggests that it was used for the distillation of aromatic oils.

The holistic tradition of Ayurvedic medicine in India is three thousand years old. It often combines the use of scented oils, spices and massage. Although it is not called aromatherapy, it is clear its practitioners are aware of the therapeutic value of certain plants and spices.

GREECE AND ROME

The way to health is to have an aromatic bath and scented massage every day.

HIPPOCRATES.

Gradually the knowledge of the oils was spreading. The Greeks passed on their knowledge to the Romans and by the time that Ovid (43 BC–AD 17) was writing his poetry, Rome and Greece had many perfume shops selling fragrant oils. 'Wives are out of fashion, mistresses are in. Rose leaves now are dated, now cinnamon's the thing' is a quote from that time that draws attention to the fashion for fragrance.

Like the Egyptians, the Greeks and Romans were also aware that the oils were beneficial. 'The best recipe for good health is to apply sweet scents to the brain' was generally the motto they lived by. Hippocrates (460–370 BC) known to many as the father of medicine, recommended the use of the oils to stem the spread of the plague and the streets of Athens were lined with fumigations burning oils to help clean the air and prevent contagious diseases spreading.

Apart from being used for disease and healing, the aromatics also provided a sensory experience. Nero is said to have had a pipe system in his house through which he could send various fragrances spraying onto his guests. Apart from the fragrance, the oils he sprayed also had the ability to alter mood (as well as cleansing the air with their antiseptic and antibacterial properties). One could speculate, knowing the oils available back then, that if Nero had wanted his guests to sleep well late at night, he could have piped marjoram for its sedative properties into the rooms of his guests, or he may have used rose for its aphrodisiac effect in order to ensure a lively evening.

It would seem that in ancient Greece and Rome the sense of smell was much more appreciated than it is today. Often, gifts of scent were taken by guests attending a dinner party in much the same way that we will take along a bottle of wine today. Scent was also an important part of festival or ceremonies. Nowadays, we tend to limit our senses to the visual, oral and aural. We use sight, taste and sound to celebrate whereas the ancients would include the sensation of fabulous aromas that could also evoke mood and ambiance.

At the games in Daphne, one of the Kings of Syria who ruled from 175–164 BC had processions of girls carrying golden bowls

of perfume to sprinkle on spectators. They were given gifts of spikenard, lily, cinnamon, saffron, frankincense and myrrh. A far cry from modern festivals where often the only aromas are those of cigarettes, traffic fumes or hot dog and hamburger stands – hardly a fragrance to uplift the senses or evoke a heady, mind-expanding experience.

In the time of Julius Caesar (100–44 BC), it was the fashion to gather socially for an aromatic bath followed by a massage. By the third century AD, Rome was bathing capital of the world.

The ancient Greeks and Romans also made liberal use of rose oil in food and wine. Known for its ability to aid digestion and the liver functions, in those days of excess this oil was much valued. The quelling effect of rose on the intoxicating effects of alcohol would allow them to drink more.

One of the most famous physicians from this time was Dioscorides. He was a Greek physician in Nero's army. He wrote the famous text book on the use of plants called *De Materea Medica* which contains a wealth of information on aromatic essences:

Myrrh: doth strengthen the teeth and gummes and is soporific.

Marjoram: soporific.

Juniper: is diuretical and if anointed about the genitall before conjunction it doth cause sterilitie.

Perhaps this use of juniper is a record of one of the world's first spermicide. Certainly marjoram is still used as a soporific and juniper as diuretic.

The fall of the Roman empire (generally dated to AD 410) signalled a decline in the level of civilization in Europe especially with regard to bathing. It seems that later the oils were used more to mask the smell of the many unwashed rather than enhance bathtime. This decline meant that most of the Roman

MIDDLE EAST

In the Middle East, in Persia in AD 980–1,037 lived a philosopher and physician called Ibn Sina, known more often as Avicenna, who is often credited with the discovery of distillation. Although there is evidence it was known of before this, it was certainly Avicenna who improved it and brought it into popular use. His book *The Canon of Medicinae* was used as a standard work for many centuries. In it, he explored the use of aromatics, medicinal plants and spices. He was also greatly in favour of the use of massage, traction and fruit fasting as part of a detoxifying diet.

> Restorative friction produces repose. Its object is to disperse effete matter formed in the muscles and not expelled by exercise. It causes the effete matter to disperse and so removes fatigue. Such friction is soft and gentle and is best done with oil or perfumed ointment.

We know today that massage can help break down uric and lactic acids that can build up to excess when a muscle is overused. Also this can be helped along by the use of oils that are detoxifying and diuretic.

It was thought that the crusading knights in the Middle Ages brought the oils and perfumes back from their travels in Egypt and Syria to Europe.

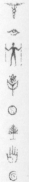

EUROPE IN THE MIDDLE AGES

THE PLAGUE

The plague hit Europe in the early fourteenth century destroying between a third and a half of the population. It was caused by bacterium transmitted by fleas borne by migrating Asian rats. So, ironically, the same ships on the trade routes that brought the herbs and spices to the West also brought the rats and fleas carrying the bubonic plague – disease and antidote on the same ship.

Just as Hippocrates had urged people to use essential oils to protect them against the plague so too did the European physicians. Doctors treating the plague used to wear protective garments, gloves and a mask which was filled with cloves, cinnamon and spices. Pomanders stuck with garlic and cloves were worn around the neck to ward off infection. (Cinnamon and clove are both antiviral and antibacterial and modern research has shown that they are particularly effective in killing off typhoid and cholera bacteria.)

Master Alexis, an alchemist of the time, wrote:

> To make a verie good perfume against the plague, you must take mastich, chypre, incense, mace, wormwood, myrrh, aloes wood, musk, ambergris, nutmegs, myrtle, bay, rosemary, sages, roses, elder, cove juniper, and pitch. All these stamped and mixed together, you shall set upon the coales and so perfume the chamber.

Sponges soaked in these oils would have offered some protection and relief to the sick but, sadly, they were too little, too late. It is interesting to note, however, that figures show that the group least affected by the plague were the perfumers who, working with the oils all day, were protected by the antiseptic properties.

Another popular mixture recommended for protection against the plague and disease was known as four thieves vinegar. Consisting of absinthe, rosemary, lavender, sage, mint, cinnamon, nutmeg, garlic, camphor in vinegar, it was applied all over to fight infection.

THE SIXTEENTH AND SEVENTEENTH CENTURIES IN EUROPE

In the sixteenth century, the Italians developed the art of perfumery. Catherine de Medici (1519–89) created a vogue for aromatic products by wearing them on her hems and on her gloves. She is also said to have dispatched a few poisonous gloves to her enemies. Much of the perfume however, as well as being used for protection was also used to hide the smell of unwashed bodies or used as an aphrodisiac. Bathing was not in vogue. Elizabeth I (1533–1603) had her cloaks and shoes treated with the oils.

In Germany, Hieronymous Braunschweig wrote a number of books on distillation. *New Volkemne Distillierbuch* in 1591 referred to 25 essential oils.

This was the time of the great herbalists in Europe – William Turner, John Gerarde, John Parkinson and William Culpeper, who in 1652 wrote:

> The oil drawn from the leaves and flowers is of sovereign help, to touch the temples and the nostrils with two to three drops for all diseases of the brain, for the inward diseases it must be done with discretion, as the case requires, for it is very quick and piercing.

In *The Treasure of Euonymus* , published in 1559, Conrad Gesner conveyed how the essential oils had the power to conserve all strengths and prolong life:

Rosemare: it strengtheneth the harte, the braine, the sinews and the hoole bodye. Members sick of the palsy it heateth them for the most part and healeth them sometimes. Fistulaes and cancars that give not place to other medicines, it healeth them through lye.

In 1616, J.J. Wecker wrote:

Perfumes are certainly compound medicine which can affect the mind and eliminate all bad odours and infections in the air that surrounds us.

THE NINETEENTH CENTURY IN EUROPE

For centuries, the knowledge of herbalism had been passed down by householders and the herbalists from generation to generation until, finally, in the nineteenth century the practice faded out as the new trend of synthetic medicine took over.

However, there was still interest in the healing power of plants in some quarters. In 1882, William Whitla wrote *Materea Medica*, another book referring to 22 oils. In 1887, the first tests were recorded to find if the oils were actually antibacterial. Chamberland in 1887 and Cadeac and Meunier in 1888 published studies revealing that micro-organisms of glandular and yellow fever were easily killed by oils, especially oil of cinnamon, thyme, lavender and juniper. Since then experts have confirmed their findings and shown that many of the oils are antibacterial, antifungal and antiviral and all of them are antiseptic.

However, this wasn't enough as the tide had turned in medicine; chemical research was now popular, the emphasis being in favour of the curative rather than the preventative. The use of medicinal plants, oils and herbs was considered outdated and old fashioned. Physicians were anxious to move forward into the next century and all the new discoveries it had to offer in the world of medicine. In their hunger for new knowledge they neglected aromatics – it was a case of throwing a baby out with the bath water.

THE TWENTIETH CENTURY

In Italy in the 1920s, Giovanni Gatti and Renato Cayola looked into the psychotherapeutic value of the oils and their action on the nervous system and found that the oils had much to offer.

Rene Gattefossé is called the father of modern aromatherapy because he was the first to call the practice of using the oils 'aromatherapy'. He published his first book, *Aromatherapie*, in 1928 followed by scientific papers and several other books largely relating to the oils. He knew that the oils had greater antiseptic properties than some of the antiseptic chemicals used at that time, a knowledge that was apparently put into practise when he burnt his hands. Plunging them into a nearby vat of lavender, he was amazed at the short time it took for his hands to heal with no sign of infection and leaving no scar. In 1939, Albert Couvner published a book detailing the medicinal application of the oils.

In a French school, Dr Sztark introduced the idea of vaporizing oils into the classroom. He'd read about how in previous centuries the oils were used this way as a preventive measuure against disease and realized it could be of great use in a school environment. Today if one person catches a virus in school or in an office, it often goes round the whole building, affecting everyone in the process. Burning preventative oils would be a sensible solution.

Dr Jean Valnet was a doctor who pioneered work with the oils and published his findings in *The Practice of Aromatherapy* in

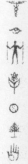

1964. He used the oils to treat wounds, burns, gangrene and in his psychiatric work with mentally disturbed patients while working as an army surgeon in Indo-China. It is thanks to him that aromatherapy is recognized pharmacologically, especially in France and Switzerland. He wrote:

> Forgotten and ignored for many years, aromatic essences are coming back into their own, for many researchers and for a large section of public opinion, as the stars of medicine. Faced with a mounting toll of complications known to have been caused by aggressively synthesized chemical medications, many patients are now unwilling to be treated except by natural therapies, foremost amongst which plants and their essences have a rightful place.

Marguerite Maury was a biochemist who studied Valnet's work. She rekindled the ancient art of combining the oils with massage and looked into the benefits of the oils for health, beauty and the effects of the oils on mood and emotion.

Robert Tisserand is the author of one of the first books in English on the subject of aromatherapy. His book, *The Art of Aromatherapy*, generated great interest in 1977 and paved the way for the growth of aromatherapy in England. In it, he wrote:

> Aromatherapy is a subject which at least in England has so far been steeped in magic and mystery. This may give it a certain amount of appeal but it also creates a great deal of confusion and misunderstanding and leaves most people in a state of relative ignorance. I hope that this book will shed some light on the subject.

Since the publication of that first book, Tisserand has been teaching and writing about the oils and his company address is given at the back of this book as one of the recommended suppliers of the oils today.

His company even does mail order and so the story has come full circle – from ancient Egypt to your doorstep.

Since *The Art of Aromotherapy*, many other books have appeared on the shelves of local bookshops, books advising on the oils for practitioners and home users alike, so bringing the practice of aromatherapy well within reach of everyone.

In 1985, the IFA, International Federation of Aromatherapists, was formed. This was made up of a small group of practitioners who wanted to ensure a standard for practising aromatherapists and suppliers of the oils. It also wanted to make certain that those calling themselves aromatherapists had received proper training. Since setting up, it has regular meetings and issues a regular newsletter.

Many other organizations have sprung up since then (many are listed at the back of the book) and there are training schools and practitioners in most major cities throughout the UK.

The AOC was formed in 1991. It is the governing body for all aromatherapists in the UK and is a member of the BCMA (British Complementary Medicine Association). It is composed of training organizations and aromatherapy associations.

This is what it says about them in their introductory pamphlet.

The AOC was formed:

1) To unify the profession.

2) To establish common standards of training and ensure that all organizations registered with the council provide appropriate standards of professional practice and conduct for their members.

3) To act as a public watchdog.

4) To provide for all organizations within aromatherapy a collective voice through which it will initiate and sustain political dialogue within government, civil and medical bodies, in order to enhance the best interests of aromatherapy.

5) To offer a mediation and arbitration service in any disputes involving aromatherapy organizations.

6) To initiate, support and sponsor research into aromatherapy.

And so, at last the practice of aromatherapy and the essential oils are getting the full attention they deserve both in the world of research where the properties and benefits of the oils are being thoroughly investigated and in the media where hardly a magazine appears nowadays without some mention of the healing powers of the oils.

The oils are also more widely available now than ever before appearing in most good health shops and many chemists around the country.

ABOUT
THE ESSENTIAL OILS

WHERE DO THE OILS COME FROM?

The oils come from locations all over the world. They are extracted from fruits, herbs, trees, roots, leaves, barks and spices, each with its own particular scent and healing property.

The following chart will tell you exactly where the essences come from:

A) Geographically.

B) Which part of the flower or plant the oil is obtained from.

1

ESSENTIAL OIL	ORIGIN	PART OF PLANT OBTAINED FROM
Angelica:	China/Egypt/England/Spain/USSR/Belgium	seed/roots
Aniseed:	Indonesia/India/North Africa/Central/ South America	seed pod
Basil:	Bulgaria/USA/Madagascar/Seychelles/Asia/ Europe	whole plant
Bay:	Jamaica/South America/Morocco/Spain	leaves

Benzoin:	Indonesia/Borneo/Thailand	tree trunk
Bergamot:	Ivory Coast/Italy/Morocco/Guinea	peel of fruit
Birch:	E.Europe/Holland/Germany/USSR	tree bark
Black Pepper:	Sri Lanka/Brazil/SE Asia/India/Indonesia/ Malaysia	berries
Cajuput:	Vietnam/Philippines/Australia	leaves/twigs
Camomile:	England/France/Hungary/Egypt/Morocco/ Bulgaria/Yugoslavia	flower/leaves
Camphor:	Borneo/Sumatra/China/Japan	wood
Caraway:	North Europe/Africa/Russia	seeds
Cardamom:	Guatamala/India/Ceylon/France/S.America	seeds
Carrot seed:	England/France/Europe/Egypt/India	root/seeds
Cedarwood:	Morocco/USA/North America	wood
Celery:	India/France	seeds
Cinnamon:	Sri Lanka/India/Madagascar	bark/twigs/ leaves
Citronella:	Sri Lanka/South America/Madagascar	grass
Clary sage:	Bulgaria/Spain/France/USSR/USA/Morocco	flowering tops
Clove:	Madagascar/Philippines/East Indies/Zanzibar/ West Indies	flower buds
Coriander:	Russia/USSR/Italy/India/USA/Tunisia/Morocco/ Mediterranean	seeds, leaves
Cumin:	Egypt/Sicily/Morocco/India/Mediterranean/Asia	seeds, fruit
Cypress:	France/Mediterranean/Germany	leaves, twigs
Dill:	Mediterranean	seeds, fruit
Elemi:	France/Mexico	tree bark
Eucalyptus:	China/Australia/Spain/Brazil/California	leaves, twigs
Fennel:	Spain/Japan/India/Russia/Mediterranean/ Romania/Northern Europe	seeds
Frankincense:	Somalia/China/Ethiopia/Lebanon/ Southern Arabia	tree bark
Galbanum:	Iran/Lebanon/Cape of Good Hope	tree bark
Garlic:	Spain/Egypt/Sicily/France	stem/pods
Geranium:	Zimbabwe/Reunion/Egypt	leaves
	China/Morocco/Algeria	stalks
	USSR/Italy/Spain	flowers

Ginger:	Nigeria/China/Japan/Java/West Africa	roots
Grapefruit:	Israel/USA/Brazil	rind of fruit
Hyssop:	France/Brazil/Palastine	leaves
	Italy	flowering tops
Jasmine:	Morocco/France/Egypt/China/Algeria/	flowers
	Morocco/Italy	
Juniper:	Tyrol/India/North Africa/North America/	berries
	North Asia/Europe	
Lavender:	France/Bulgaria/Yugoslavia/England/Tasmania	flowering tops
Lemon:	Spain/Brazil/Israel/USA/Argentina	fruit rind
Lemongrass:	Cochin/Brazil/Sri Lanka/Central Africa/China	whole plant
Lime:	West Indies/Brazil/Mexico/Italy	fruit rind
Linden Blossom:	France/England	flowers
Mandarin:	Brazil/Spain/Italy/China/Argentina/California	rind of fruit
Marjoram:	Spain/Egypt/Hungary/	leaves
	France/Germany/Portugal	flowering tops
Melissa:	Tanzania/Europe/Mediterranean	leaves
Myrrh:	Somalia/Ethiopia/North Africa	tree bark/resin
Myrtle:	Morocco, Austria/Tunisia	leaves
Neroli:	Tunisia/France/Egypt/Italy/Morocco/Portugal	flowers
Niaouli:	Madagascar/Australia/East Indies	twigs and leaves
Nutmeg:	Indonesia/West Indies	seed
Orange:	Brazil/France/Spain/USA/Israel	fruit rind
Origanum:	North Africa/Europe	leaves
	Asia/Egypt	flowering tops
Palmarosa:	Madagascar/Brazil/Comora Islands/	whole plant
	Central America	
Parsley:	Europe	seeds
Patchouli:	Indonesia/China/Japan/Madagascar/Paraguay	leaves
Peppermint:	England/America/China/Europe	whole plant
Petitgrain:	Paraguay/France/Italy/Brazil	leaves/twigs
Pimento:	West Indies/India/Reunion	berries/twigs
Pine:	Siberia/Europe/USSR/North America	needles/twigs

PRINCIPLES OF AROMATHERAPY

Rose:	Morocco/Bulgaria/Turkey/France	flowers/petals
Rosemary:	Spain/Tunisia/Zimbabwe/France/Japan/ Yugoslavia	flowers/leaves
Rosewood:	Brazil	wood
Sage:	China/Mediterranean/Yugoslavia	flowers/leaves
Sandalwood:	East India/Indonesia	wood
Spearmint:	USA/China/Europe	flowering tops
	Mediterranean/Russia	leaves
Tangerine:	Brazil/China/USA/Sicily	peel of fruit
Tarragon:	Russia/France	flowering plant
Thyme:	Zimbabwe/Egypt/Mediterranean	leaves
	Gt Britain/America/France	flowering tops
Tea tree:	Australia/Tasmania	leaves/twigs
Verbena:	Algeria/Spain/South America	stalks and leaves
Vetivert:	Indonesia/Philippines/Comora Islands	roots
Violet:	Italy/France/England/Greece/Egypt	leaves
Yarrow:	Europe/Africa/USA	flowering tops
	Western Asia	leaves
Ylang-ylang:	Comora Islands/Indonesia/Phillipines/Seychelles	flowers

WHAT ARE ESSENTIAL OILS?

Essential oils are the aromatic substances extracted from the part of the plant that gives its individual characteristics of scent, colour and healing components. Some have likened this to the soul or life-force of the plant, others describe it as the hormone of the plant, others say it is the DNA. Whatever the description, it is that part of the plant that gives us the whole, shaping its unique makeup and medicinal properties.

Some plants may yield more than one oil, for example the orange blossom tree gives us three different oils. It gives neroli from the flowers, orange from the fruit peel and petitgrain from the leaves and twigs. Each of these three oils have a different scent and different use. Neroli, apart from its pleasing scent, is very calming and can be used to help lower blood pressure. It is also wonderful for skincare. Orange is good for aiding digestion and constipation and petitgrain is good for use in convalescence and often used for insomnia.

ARE THE PLANTS PICKED AT A PARTICULAR TIME OF YEAR?

Every one is different. It isn't just a question of going out, getting the plant or flower at any time of the year and extracting the oil. Collecting the plant parts at the right time is an art in itself. For example:

Pepper oil: is collected from unripe berries

Coriander oil: when the fruit is ripe

Jasmine: flowers are picked at night and before the flower is one day old.

Sandalwood: is extracted when the tree is 30 years old and 30 feet high.

Ylang-ylang: flowers are picked early morning when the scent is at its strongest.

Juniper: must first be dried before being distilled.

Rose: is best processed at the source so as not to lose any of the oil.

As with grapes, where there are good and bad harvests which in turn affect the wines of a particular year, in the same way the purity and scent of an oil can depend on various factors such as weather, harvest and time of picking. Oils extracted from plants grown in a natural environment where the air is pure and the climate perfect, are obviously going to be a better quality than plants grown say, in a field in a polluted climate near a busy motorway with lots of traffic fumes.

WHAT ARE THE CONSTITUENTS OF THE OILS?

Each oil has a different molecular structure which gives it its individuality. It is this that gives each oil its unique scent and individual therapeutic properties. The components are made up from:

Alcohols: menthol, linalol, geranol, nerol, borneol.

Aldehydes: citral, benzoic, citronella, vanilline.

Acids: cinnamic, benzoic.

Phenols: eugenol, thymol.

Esters; benzyl, linalyl.

Acetones: cineol, jasmone, irone.

Terpenes: pinene, camphene, terpineol, phellandrene, limonene.

Each oil has a complex chemical makeup and a unique combination of the constituents. Eucalyptus for example, is made up from 250 different constituents making it virtually impossible to create synthetically and although the aroma may be simulated chemically, it could never recreate the healing power of the pure essence.

- The oils come in small dark glass bottles and are sold in their concentrate form usually in quantities of 10 or 20 ml.

- As the oils are extracted from different parts of the plant, they vary in colour and intensity. Some are brown, some are gold, some are rich red, some green yellow, some are colourless. For example, the ones extracted from flowering tops such as geranium or lavender tend to be light and almost see-through whereas the oils taken from tree bark and wood such as sandalwood or benzoin are thicker, darker, almost gum-like.

- Even though they are called essential oils, whilst still in their concentrate form, they are not, in fact, oily. They are extremely volatile and the sign of a pure essential oil is one that if spilt onto blotting-paper, it will in time disappear completely, leaving no 'greasy' mark at all.

- The most obvious way to recognize an essential oil though, is by the smell. Each of them has a unique scent and after using them for a short time, the newcomer will be able to judge for themselves which oil is which by simply removing the top of the bottle.

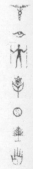

Some of the oils have a very pleasant scent: rose, neroli, rosewood, petitgrain, jasmine, ylang-ylang.

Some smell of menthol: eucalyptus, peppermint, niaouli, cajuput.

Some smell woody: sandalwood, rosewood, cedarwood.

Some smell of citrus: orange, lime, lemon, grapefruit, bergamot.

Some smell herby: rosemary, basil, thyme, clary sage, juniper, fennel.

Some spicy: cinnamon, ginger, black pepper, clove.

Some smell of disinfectant: tea tree.

Some smell completely unique and the scent is difficult to describe: frankincense, myrrh, cypress.

HOW ARE THEY EXTRACTED FROM THE PLANTS?

As the oils come from a variety of plants, trees and flowers, different methods of extraction are used. For example some produce greater quantities of oil (lavender, rosemary, tea tree), while others are more delicate and are harder to come by (rose, jasmine). These sorts of factors can determine which method is best.

DISTILLATION

This is the method most commonly used to obtain the oil. Steam is passed through vats filled with the selected part of the plant. This causes the oils to vaporize. When the steam cools, the oil has separated and can easily be collected.

SOLVENT EXTRACTION

It is similar to steam distillation in that the plant parts are placed in vats but instead of water being steamed through, volatile solvents are used. The solvents are saturated with the essential oil, and then filtered to obtain the oil. However, this method is frowned upon by some suppliers as the essential oils left behind sometimes also contain chemical residue from the solvents. However, as time moves on, more efficient and environmentally friendly solvents are being developed. It is the solvents that left the chemical residue which have up until recently, marred the reputation of oils extracted this way.

ENFLEURAGE/MACERATION

The flowers' heads are placed in layers of purified fat or wax. They are left until the oil is saturated with the perfume. The process is then repeated. The oil is then obtained either by separating the aromatic substances from the fat with a solvent or alcohol or by putting them through a centrifuge and distilling them at very low temperatures.

The result of this process is called an absolute. It can be a lengthy and complicated process which explains why the oils obtained by this method are more expensive. This method is now becoming more and more obsolete as it takes so long; it was used mainly for flowers such as jasmine, rose or neroli as the heat and pressure used in methods such as distillation could destroy the essential oil.

PRESSING

This is used for obtaining the oils from citrus fruits, lime, lemon, orange, grapefruit and tangerine. Machines are used to simply squeeze the oils from the rinds of the fruit.

WHAT ARE THE PROPERTIES OF THE OILS?

All the oils are antiseptic. Others are analgesic, antibiotic, antiviral, antispasmodic, antibacterial, antifungal, aphrodisiac, balsamic, diuretic, detoxifying, emmenagogue, expectorant, laxative, sedative, revitalizing, tonic, or vulnerary, to name some of the properties. (See appendices for a complete list.)

WHAT ARE THE BENEFITS?

One of the truly remarkable things about the oils is their ability to alter the way a person feels whilst also treating a physical complaint. Many clients will say that the day after an aromatherapy treatment, they feel in a particulary good mood or that they feel uplifted. This is because the benefits of the oils can be experienced on many levels:

- Physical complaints can be treated: stomach upset, headaches, bronchitis, sprains, backache, cellulite.

- Emotional moods lifted: depression, grief, resentment.

- Mental states: fatigue, lack of concentration, flagging memory.

The oils can be used to greater and lesser degrees to treat just about every ailment there is from stress, to cellulite, to constipation. In nature, for every nettle there is a dock leaf, so for every complaint or disorder, there is an oil that can assist in alleviating it. (For the full index of oils and their uses, see appendices.)

HOW DO THE OILS WORK?

The oils work in two ways.

1) By entering the system via the skin through massage, through the lining of the lungs through inhalation or vaporization or through the digestive system when taken orally (although this method is not advised without supervision from a trained aromatherapist).

   The oils are then absorbed into the blood stream. Once

in the system, the medicinal properties of the oils can start to do their work be it as a balsamic, antifungal or antibacterial. Sceptics may question how it can be that something that you simply breathe in can be effective in fighting disease. Yet think of the negative effects of the viruses or germs that circulate in our towns and cities: they get into our system simply through the air we breathe – flu causing even the healthiest person to take to their bed. Essential oils can be just as potent but in a positive way, they can help fight whatever is diseased in the system and are enormously effective in bringing relief. Micheline Arcier mentions in her book on aromatherapy that as part of a laboratory test a pig's head was rubbed with the essential oil of lavender. Twenty-five minutes later, the essential oil was traced to the animal's kidneys. Other tests have shown that garlic oil rubbed into the feet can later be smelt on the breath.

2) Through the aroma. We are tremendously affected by smell yet it is a sense we rarely credit. Bad smells of staleness or decay can repulse us, warning us that whatever smells that way is not good. In fact, when people are ill, their body often emits a particular odour and many doctors are aware that something is amiss by the smell of acid or slightly rotten scent. In the same way, goodness and health smells, the scent of newly baked bread, freshly cut grass, the heady perfume of jasmine on a warm summer's night, tell us whatever smells that way is alive and good.

Each essential oil has its own particular scent and affect, some uplift, some soothe, some are refreshing, some are medicinal. The scent of the oils affects the limbic system in the brain via the olfactory tract. Scent affects the autonomic nervous system

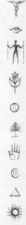

and our hormonal system. These systems govern heart rate, anger, fear, stress and memory. Just think how a scent can take you back vividly to a time or place long-forgotten. A particular perfume recalls a person just as clearly as any photograph. Smell is evocative and this is the power of the oils as each has a different scent which can evoke a reaction in us.

People often comment that certain oils smell 'clean' or 'refreshing' or as though there was 'goodness' in it. In fact, some aromatherapists let clients choose their oils by seeing which they are attracted to. Often without knowing which oil is used for what, clients will be drawn to the scent of the oil that is best for their condition. For example, people with a chest complaint are often attracted to the menthol scents as these are the ones that help relieve congestion.

METHODS OF APPLICATION

There are several ways of applying the oils.

MASSAGE

This is perhaps the most popular method of applying the oils, it is certainly the most pleasurable.

The object in applying the oils through massage is, apart from easing tension held in the body and improving the circulation, to get the oils into the system so they can start to do their work.

A different blend of oils is mixed depending on a person's particular need. By way of the massage, the oils enter into the blood stream through the skin. As it can take from six to eight hours for the oils to be completely absorbed, clients are advised not to shower for some time after an aromatherapy massage or the full benefits can be lost. What gives an aromatherapy massage that added extra apart from the pleasurable sensation of the scent, is the fact that the oils continue working long after the physical massage has finished.

It is important, however, that the oils are diluted before they are applied to the skin during the treatment. If the oils were to be used in their concentrate form straight onto the skin, they would cause a reaction; the solution would be too strong even for the most weatherbeaten, tough, insensitive skin. The sensation caused would be of burning or severe stinging. For this reason, the oils are always put into what is called carrier or base oils.

CARRIER OILS

Any one of the following oils would serve as a base oil to dilute the essential oils. It is always best to use cold pressed oils as they are the purest.

- Grapeseed: from grape seeds, the oil is a pale yellowy green and is a popular choice as it is easily available and has a medium texture liked by most people.

- Almond: from almond nuts. It is light in texture and a clear pale yellow, it is slightly more expensive but is very kind to the skin and good quality almond oil has the most wonderful scent.

- Apricot kernel: particularly good for use on the face and neck as it is very light and is easily absorbed. It tends to be one of the more expensive carriers.

- Sunflower: another popular choice for body massage as it is easy to find and contains vitamin E which is good for the skin.

- Soya: from the soya bean plant is especially good for oily skins and is easily absorbed.

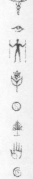

PRINCIPLES OF AROMATHERAPY

- Avocado: extracted form the avocado, this is slightly more expensive and is very rich. Containing vitamins A and B it acts as an excellent skin softener, favoured by those with dry skin.

- Wheatgerm: from the germ of the wheat, contains vitamin E and is very good for dry skin though it is often thought to be too rich in texture and smell. It can be used in combination with another lighter oil to prolong the time an oil can be used.

- Sesame: from the seeds is richer than some of the other oils and with a slight nutty aroma, like wheatgerm, it is best used in combination with other lighter oils.

Usually about a tablespoon of base oil is sufficient for a whole body massage. The base oil is put in a pot or small cup and the aromatherapy oils are added. Usually no more than three different oils are used in one session. And of those three essential oils, no more than 6 to 8 drops in total are added to the base oil.

Base oils containing lanolin are best avoided for aromatherapy as lanolin doesn't absorb through the skin and can cause a reaction on people with sensitive skins.

AROMATIC BATH

This is the easiest method of using the oils. Simply add 6 to 8 drops into your bathwater, preferentially when running the hot water as the heat will help release the scent so permeating the room as you bathe. Swish the oil around the water, as it is not soluble in water you need to disperse it as well as possible. If it all floats in one place on top of the water, it can sting the skin slightly. If it is well dispersed this won't happen and the oil will penetrate the skin without irritation.

As only part of the essential oil diffuses in the water, much of it is left floating on the surface, so much of the benefit is in the oil vaporized with the heat and breathed in, so entering the system through the lungs. As the aroma is taken in with inhalation, it will be absorbed through the lining of the lung into the blood stream.

Certain oils are not advisable for use in the bath, for example cinnamon, ginger, black pepper, thyme, sage, peppermint and eucalyptus can all sting slightly if they come directly into contact with the skin. All the oils will sting if used to excess so it is important not to put too much in.

Baths can be taken to stimulate or relax, for example a bath with bergamot, rosemary or basil in the morning would refresh whereas a soothing bath in the evening with marjoram, camomile, lavender or rosewood would help unwind and relax ready for a good night's sleep.

INHALATION

This method is particularly effective for sinus trouble, coughs, sore throats, colds, flu and any chest problems but could just as easily be used to clear a foggy head on a sluggish morning.

There are several oils which help alleviate any symptoms of congestion in the nose, sinuses or chest: eucalyptus, cajuput, niaouli, sandalwood, pine and tea tree, the latter being gentle to inhale whilst also being very potent.

This method is very useful as a preventative, especially if a virus or flu is going round. For instance, eucalyptus is antiviral and could therefore kill any germinating bug before it gets a chance to get hold.

There are two ways you can use the oils for inhalation:

A) Simply fill a bowl with boiling water, add a couple of drops of oil. Put a towel over your head and breathe deeply into the steam, coming up for air when you need.

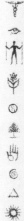

PRINCIPLES OF AROMATHERAPY

B) Purchase a steam inhaler. Many chemists stock them now and they cost around £25. You add a small amount of water, the inhaler then electrically heats it. Wait until it is steaming, then add 3 to 4 drops of essential oil and placing your nose in the bowl provided, breathe deeply. The advantage of the electric steam inhaler is that it keeps the heat from the steam coming consistently so if you have to keep coming up for air, when you go back to the machine, the water won't have cooled down.

As the aroma from the essential oil is at its most potent when released with the heat, the steam inhaler can be a good investment for getting through the winter without any coughs, colds, flu and chest complaints.

COMPRESS

This method is usually used when the oils are needed to focus on a particular area such as a sprained ankle or menstrual cramps. A compress is simply a piece of bandage, flannel or cloth that has been immersed in water containing essential oil. The compress can be hot or cold depending on the need. For a sprain, a cold compress would be soothing, using an oil to help prevent swelling and relieve pain. For a condition such as menstrual cramps a hot compress would probably be preferable. Camomile oil would be a good choice for both as it is an analgesic, relieving cramps or swelling. The cloth is applied to the part of the body in need and left there for as long as feels comfortable.

VAPORIZER

This means to use heat to release the oils into the atmosphere. This can be done by:

1) Leaving a bowl of water to which essential oils have been added near a radiator, the heat from the radiator will help release the scent into the room.

2) Many aromatherapy suppliers are now selling burners. These are usually made of pottery and have two shelves. They are no bigger than a small vase. On the lower shelf is room for a small night light, on the top shelf is a small ledge for oil. When the candle is lit, the heat from it causes the oils to permeate the atmosphere.

3) Saturate a small towel in water, wring it out then shake 6 to 8 drops of essential oil onto the towel. Drape the towel on a radiator, as the towel dries, the room will be filled with the scent of the oil.

Any one of these methods could be used to create atmosphere and aroma or to protect the air we breathe. It would be an ideal method to use in all walks of life from hospitals, doctors waiting rooms, offices and schools in fact anywhere where people are coming into contact with germs. Many people I know burn oils in this way in sick rooms if a family member or friend is unwell. Apart from creating a pleasant smell for the person who is ill (as sickrooms often get stuffy), it also protects people coming into the room from whatever virus or germ the ill person has.

AIR FRESHENER

Some people add a few drops of essential oil to lukewarm water in a water spray then simply spray it around the room for freshness and scent. Pine, lemon and lemongrasss are popular choices to use in this way keeping the air both fragrant and bacteria free.

When the oils are taken this way they are always diluted either in warm water or alcohol then simply swallowed. However, this method is not advisable without the supervision of a fully qualified practitioner. The wrong dosage can cause a severe reaction and the other methods are equally as effective and safer.

ARE THERE TIMES WHEN THE OILS SHOULDN'T BE USED?

Definitely.

1) Always dilute the oils. They should never be used for massage in their concentrate form as they will burn or sting the skin. Dilute them in a base oil such as sunflower, grapeseed or almond first. The only exceptions are lavender or tea tree which can be applied neat to burns and cuts.

2) Don't take them orally as the wrong oil or wrong amount can cause a severe reaction. Check with a practitioner who has been properly trained and is a member of one of the organizations approved of by the AOC. (For details of the AOC see appendices.) The wrong amount can cause vomiting, irritate the stomach lining and in the case of some oils, cause seizures.

3) Be careful during pregnancy. Certain oils are emmenagogue and could cause miscarriage. (See Chapter 10 for details of which these oils are.)

4) Don't put the oils close to the eyes as they can sting.

5) The following oils have been known to cause a reaction particularly in those who have a sensitive skin: sage,

cinnamon, clove, ginger, peppermint, basil, fennel, lemon grass, rosemary, thyme. The oils can be used on people with sensitive skin but in extremely reduced dosages.

6) People who suffer from epilepsy should avoid: fennel, hyssop, rosemary and wormwood. These oils can induce a fit if the wrong amount is used.

7) If suffering from hepatitis, Parkinson's disease, diphtheria or cancer only use the aromatherapy oils with the full knowledge and consent of your doctor.

8) If taking homoeopathic medicine, check with your homoeopath before using the oils as some of the oils negate the effects of homoeopathy. Particularly avoid camphor, peppermint, black pepper and eucalyptus.

9) For use on children reduce the amounts used to one per cent in a dilution.

10) Keep the oils away from young children and pets.

11) If in doubt, speak with a fully trained aromatherapist.

HOW DO I KNOW WHICH OILS TO USE AS THERE ARE SO MANY?

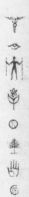

Many people coming into contact with the oils for the first time feel slightly overwhelmed by the choice of oils and the fact that one oil can help so many conditions. For example for rheumatism, you have the choice of rosemary, cypress, lavender, camomile, bay, marjoram to name but a few. It can leave a newcomer thinking what? All of them? Or one of them?

Which is most beneficial for which particular case? The fact is many of the oils are versatile and could all be of help. However, there tend to be a number that are in more common

PRINCIPLES OF AROMATHERAPY

usage than others. Often this is because one of many reasons:

1) They are easily available, for example lavender and rosemary are easy to obtain as they grow in great abundance and are easy to extract through distillation.

2) They are cheaper than other oils. For example fennel, lemongrass or rose (amongst others) could all be used for indigestion. Rose can cost £20-£25 for just 5 ml. Lemongrass or fennel however would cost under £5 for 10 ml. All three oils would be of benefit, just because the rose is more expensive doesn't mean it is more effective. It is more expensive because it is harder to obtain. I would save the rose for special cases where no other oil would work as an alternative such as grief after the death of a loved one or as a luxury in a skin preparation where it is particularly effective.

3) A particular scent is preferred. Juniper and fennel are both excellent diuretics yet some people find the strong smell of fennel too overwhelming and so would pick juniper. As you become familiar with the oils and their individual aromas, you will find that you too start to favour certain oils to the exclusion of others.

HOW DO I STORE THE OILS?

1) Keep them away from heat and direct sunlight preferably in a cool place. Some people keep them in the fridge which definitely does prolong their life, however when you come to use them you may find they have thickened slightly and will need a little time to thaw before they pour easily form the bottle.

2) Store them in glass bottles as they are potent substances and can melt plastic.

3) Keep them labelled. It takes some time to acquaint yourself with the oils purely by their scent and as the bottles often become oily with regular use, the labels can slide off leaving you with the dilemma of trying to remember what smelt like what!

4) Replace the tops as the oils are affected by oxygen, light, heat and moisture. These factors will determine an oils 'shelf' life. Most oils will last up to two years if kept in a fridge.

5) Once an oil has been diluted into a carrier oil, it will only last for a few months. Storing it in the fridge will help it last longer.

If kept with care, most of the oils can last up to a year. Oils that are past their usage date will smell slightly rancid.

It is advisable in the beginning to buy oils in small quantities. As you experiment, you'll discover which aromas you prefer, which are obviously going to be used a lot depending on an individual or family's requirement and which are going to remain at the back of the box unused and hardly touched.

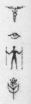

THE OILS AND YOU: FINDING A PRACTITIONER OR CHOOSING HOME USE

When it comes to benefiting from the use of the oils, you have two choices:

1) Find a local practitioner and have regular treatments.

2) Learn about how to use the oils for yourself.

GOING FOR TREATMENT

HOW DO I FIND A GOOD PRACTITIONER?

Through the AOC (Aromatherapy Organizations Council). The AOC was set up amongst other things 'to provide appropriate standards of professional practice and conduct for their members. And act as a public watchdog'. They monitor the standard of practising aromatherapists, this is to protect the reputation of practitioners as well as members of the public looking for treatment. Simply write to the AOC asking for their general information booklet and enclosing an SAE. The address is at the back in the appendices. The booklet they send back to you will contain a recent list of all the associations in the AOC plus a number of training schools. Some of the schools aren't listed in the booklet as there so many; however, as long as a school is affiliated with one of the AOC approved associations, (all the associations are listed) it will have AOC approval.

You can contact any of the associations and ask for a list of approved practitioners. There are so many now, all over the country, you should easily be able to find one within a convenient distance.

WHAT QUALIFICATIONS SHOULD I LOOK FOR?

An aromatherapist who is:

1) A member of one of the AOC affiliated associations, all of which are listed at the back of their information booklet or who has trained at an AOC approved training school.

2) Fully insured to practise. They should be able to show proof of such if you ask.

As the oils are so easily available, someone who can do basic massage can buy a few of the oils and call themselves an aromatherapist. They may be well trained in massage or beauty therapy but they are not qualified to call themselves aromatherapists unless they have done the proper training. This is why it is always safest to check that someone claiming to do aromatherapy actually has the relevant qualifications.

A properly trained aromatherapist will have the complete set of between 20 and 40 different oils and will mix up a completely unique blend of oils for each individual client she treats. Her training will have taught her about the contraindications, which oils can have adverse reactions, how to blend oils correctly, what amounts, which oils are best for various conditions amongst other things. It is not a training completed in an weekend. Most courses take up to a year full-time, two years part-time with an examination to pass at the end before they can call themselves an aromatherapist.

Some beauty salons and even some health clubs are supplied with three or four basic aromatherapy mixes which they offer when a client goes for an aromatherapy treatment. One is for relaxation, one for revitalization and then either one for cellulite or for sport massage.

The difference between having three ready mixed oils and 30 or so individual oils is that if someone goes for treatment to a qualified practitioner, she will mix up a unique blend which is going to be more helpful to the individual than a readymade mix that is used on everybody. For example, someone may go for a treatment because they are having trouble relaxing. There are many reasons why this might be which in turn will cause different symptoms:

- emotional grief, in which case rose would help

- muscular strain as a result of bad posture or sports injury, in which case rosemary and ginger would be good

- trouble sleeping, in which case a soporific such as marjoram would be best

- deep anxiety, which melissa could help

- headaches would be relieved with peppermint or lavender

- eczema can be a result of stress in which case lavender, camomile, geranium or juniper would help bring relief

- backache

- mental fatigue

The list is long as every client's needs are different depending on their circumstances and lifestyle. In each case, if with a trained practitioner, a different blend of oils would be used.

The choice of combinations is therefore complex.

The standard relaxation oil blend used in many salons often does contain aromatherapy oils and they can give a very pleasant massage. However, what a client is paying a bit extra for when they seek help from someone claiming to be an aromatherapist is the training in the art of mixing the right blend for a particular individual's condition and need at a particular time. People without the proper qualifications would be more honest if they were to advertise massage with aromatherapy oils rather than aromatherapy.

Most aromatherapists are well aware of the importance of winning the public's trust when it comes to practising and most have made sure that they are on one of the approved lists.

WHAT ACTUALLY HAPPENS IN AN AROMATHERAPY SESSION?

At the first session, the aromatherapist will start by filling in a questionnaire. This is to:

A) Take your details for their records.

B) To find out if there's anything in your medical history that they should be made aware of: any allergies, conditions, past problems or sensitivities. This is to help them build up a picture of your background but also to alert them to any contraindications, for example, if you had diabetes or epilepsy or were pregnant, precautions would be taken in choosing oils.

C) Learn about your lifestyle. Your job, your diet, your sleep patterns. All these will help them when it comes to selecting what oils are going to be best for you.

D) Discover the reason for seeking treatment. Have you come

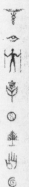

with a particular complaint that needs attending to, for help in relaxation or simply for the pure pleasure of the experience.

E) Some may ask for your doctor's details as with your permission they may wish to inform your GP that you are receiving treatment.

F) To keep a record of which oils were used on which date and the treatment given.

After the practitioner has taken your details, you will be asked to take off your clothes and lie on a couch where you will be covered in towels. Aromatherapists know that not everyone likes showing their body and are careful to preserve clients' modesty by keeping the parts of the body that aren't being worked on covered in towels.

After the practitioner has mixed a blend of oils for you into the carrier oil, she will apply it to your body through massage. Some start with the back, some with the feet, but in the course of the treatment, oil is applied to the whole body through the various strokes of massage.

Don't feel that you have to make conversation. It is not a social occasion and most people usually get most out of it if they just let go to the experience and drift off into an hour of scented relaxation. You have nothing to do but lie back and enjoy the sensation.

When the massage is over, you are usually left to lie for a few minutes and told to get up when you feel ready. As it can take four to eight hours for the oils to be absorbed into the bloodstream, clients are advised to wait for that time before they bath or shower otherwise the full benefit will be lost. At the end of a session, the practitioner may suggest further sessions or make some recommendations for use of the oils at home, advising oils for the bath or for inhalation depending on your condition. They may also make comments about your lifestyle. For example, some will suggest dietary changes when treating cellulite or gentle exercise to help a stiff back.

HOW LONG DOES A SESSION LAST?

Most aromatherapy sessions last between an hour and an hour and a half, although sometimes practitioners will see clients for half an hour. If you can go for a full hour, it is more beneficial as many people take about twenty minutes before they relax, and if they've just booked for half an hour, it can feel as if it's all over too soon.

WHEN IS THE BEST TIME TO GO FOR A TREATMENT?

A treatment is best booked when there are no immediate appointments or demands straight after. This is:

1) For maximum benefit, it is good to relax and let the body and mind have some time to enjoy the sensation of unwinding. If you have to immediately whizz back into fast gear, dashing to a next appointment, some of the good feeling can go unappreciated.

2) People can feel a bit drowsy after a session (particularly after the first session). The oils are potent and can stop you in your tracks. So often people put how they feel on the back burner and rise to the many demands made on them day to day. An aromatherapy session can put a person back in touch with how they really are so it's always advisable to try and book a session on a day when not to much is going to be demanded of you afterwards.

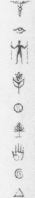

HOW OFTEN SHOULD
SOMEONE HAVE TREATMENTS?

This can depend on several factors, the urgency of a condition, the need and the bank balance. Some people make it a regular part of their lifestyle and have regular sessions booked in advance every week or fortnight. Others go every month, others book a series of treatments when the need is felt, others just go every now and then. It will help in all cases as a little is better than none at all.

As aromatherapy works as a preventative, a client with a particular weakness would be advised to book regular sessions even if it's only every eight weeks. For example, for someone in a high stress job, a regular aromatherapy can help keep any minor disorders building into major ones.

A client with a particular problem may be advised to book several treatments in a short space of time until the condition has cleared up or has been significantly relieved. For example, if someone was suffering from headaches or migraine due to temporary pressures, it is unlikely that one session would 'fix' it. However, after a series of sessions, the aromatherapist will have been able to undo much of the tension that was building and causing the headaches.

Lastly, you don't have to feel stressed or ill to go. Many people simply go when they feel like being pampered as there is no doubt it is an extremely pleasurable as well as beneficial treatment. They can enjoy the knowledge that as well as being pampered they are also taking care of their health.

WHAT WILL IT COST?

This will vary according to the town and the practitioner. It can cost from £20 to £45 for an hour to an hour and a half session. Some practitioners do home visits and obviously charge more for this service.

Most practitioners include the price of oils in the price but some charge for them separately so it's always best to check beforehand. As some of the oils are very expensive, for instance if a practitioner uses jasmine, you may find that you are asked to pay for it at the end.

ARE ALL AROMATHERAPY TREATMENTS THE SAME?

No. For two reasons.

1) Each aromatherapist has their own personality, manner and often extra qualifications. Even if two practitioners have done the same training, their treatments may feel very different because everyone brings their own particular touch to it. Some are very gentle, others prefer to do deeper tissue work.

   Many aromatherapists carry on their training in body-work and you will find many practising aromatherapists are also trained in reflexology, shiatsu, lymphatic drainage, facial or sports massage. All this will add to their skills and ability to treat you. It can do no harm to try a few in your area until you find one with whom you feel completely comfortable, whose personality suits you and whose methods you prefer. A recommendation from people you know is often a good sign.

2) As your requirements change, so the practitioner will adjust your treatment and the oils she uses. One session, she may physically pay particular attention to your back, another time to your neck. One session she may use oils to relax you and by the end of the session you may feel ready for bed, another time you may need revitalizing and so she'll use oils leaving you feeling refreshed and ready to face the day.

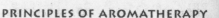

HOW TO USE THE OILS YOURSELF/ AROMATHERAPY ON A BUDGET

Although an aromatherapy treatment with a qualified practitioner is both pleasurable and beneficial, sadly many of the people who need the treatment most have either not got the time or the money. This needn't be an obstacle.

Learning the basic elements of the massage and the use of the oils can be one of the best investments you could ever make to help children, friends and partners. There are three ways you can do this.

MASSAGE COURSES/SCHOOLS

Many establishments now run weekend courses on aromatherapy and many adult education centres also run classes both during the day and in the evening. People can attend and learn the basics and any do's and don'ts for home use.

Details can be found in:

A) Your local library which will hold details of the adult education centres with dates, times and costs.

B) Local health shops and centres often have notice boards with details of any weekend courses run by local aromatherapists.

C) Local papers are another place to look for advertisements of short-term classes.

D) At the back of the book are details of all AOC training courses, some of which are full-time, some are part-time. Many people attend with no intention of actually setting up in practice, they just want to know as much about the oils as they can for their own use at home. The Tisserand

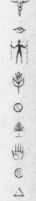

Institute for example, as well as running diploma courses for those who want to do aromatherapy as a career, also regularly runs weekend seminars for anyone who wants to learn the basics for use at home and for first aid.

VIDEOS AVAILABLE

For those who haven't the time for courses no matter how short, there is a video available from WH Smith's called *Shirley Price's Aromatherapy and Massage*. It shows you how to do a simple massage, and explains what the essential oils are and how they work. It also shows you how to blend and mix the oils for a number of common ailments such as headaches, stress, insomnia, menstrual pain and arthritis.

There are also other videos available that teach you massage methods. If you follow this book's instructions on mixing and applying the oils, these videos can take you through different stages of a massage step by step until you feel confident enough to do it without the video accompanying you.

LEARNING ABOUT THE OILS FROM BOOKS

The next chapter details which oils are most useful to have for home use. They can be used at home in the variety of ways mentioned in Chapter 3:

A) For inhalation in winter when the family have coughs, colds or blocked sinuses.

B) For vaporization.

C) In aromatic baths. Familiarize yourself with the oils that are safe for home use and those which can irritate the skin and any contraindications (See Chapter 3). If used properly, the essential oils can be used by all the family to great advantage. Relaxing baths of camomile or lavender can be taken after a hard day's work, revitalizing baths of bergamot and rosemary in the morning, detoxifying baths of juniper for hangovers.

D) Massage.

PREPARING TO DO A MASSAGE

What you need are:

A) A warm room. It is important that whoever is to be massaged feels comfortable as it is hard to relax when you have taken your clothes off and are shivering with the cold. Also body temperature drops when you are lying still, so ensure that the heating is adequate.

B) Warm the towels you are going to use. If you have radiators in the room, keep towels warm on them, it adds to the feeling of being cared for and the relaxation and luxuriousness of the experience.

C) A flat surface where the person being massaged can lie comfortably and where there is room for you to get round without restriction.

D) Soft lighting. No one wants to turn over to the brash glare of a 200 watt light bulb above them. If you haven't got side lights that can be dimmed, invest in some candles, but place them safely out of your way as you don't want to knock them over as you move around.

E) Background music (if desired). Many people find it helps them to switch off if they have some gentle music to distract them from stressful thoughts of how they're going to pay next month's mortgage payment or what they've got to do at work the next day. Let them choose the music as they may not like your taste.

F) A selection of essential oils, a carrier oil in which to dilute them and a small bowl in which to mix them.

Finally, switch phones onto answering machine and take the time to be undisturbed, next week it may be your turn.

WHERE CAN I BUY THE OILS?

As aromatherapy becomes more popular, the oils are more widely available and are on sale locally in many good chemists and health shops. You will also find you can buy many ready-made aromatherapy products from skincare creams, to hair shampoos and bath lotions.

If you are in doubt about the quality of products sold, the suppliers listed in the appendices do a mail order service for oils and beauty preparations as well. They only supply pure, unadulterated authentic essential oils of the highest quality. You can contact them for a price list for oils in their concentrate form and you will find that they also sell carrier oils, oil burners plus a whole range of natural beauty products from skincare to soap and bath oils.

HOW MUCH DO THE OILS COST?

The chart below is to give you an idea of what you can expect to pay for individual oils. It is an average price list based on a few different suppliers' price lists for the public at the time the lists were published.

If you look you will see the oils vary quite considerably in price for the same amount. For example, eucalyptus and lemon are much cheaper to buy than say, jasmine or neroli. This does not mean that the cheaper oils are less valuable therapeutically, simply that they are more readily available as they are easier to

56

obtain and extract. If you use this as a gauge, it will also help you decide whether the oils you are buying are the genuine article. For instance, I would expect to pay anything from £15 to £40 for only 5 ml of rose absolute or rose otto and about £4–5 for 10 ml of lavender. If I was charged £3 for the rose and £20 for the lavender, I would question the supplier.

Also take note that the prices quoted here are mainly per 10 ml. Often the oils are sold in 5, 10, 20, 50, or 100 ml and obviously the price will vary on the amount. I haven't listed every single essential oil, only the ones in common usage.

- You will find that organic oils tend to be more expensive.

2

PRICE GUIDE FROM AUTUMN 1995

ESSENTIAL OIL	AMOUNT	PRICE
Basil:	10ml	£6.50
Benzoin:	10ml	£3.70
Bergamot:	10ml	£6.00
Black Pepper:	10ml	£6.20
Cajuput:	10ml	£4.50
Cardoman:	5ml	£8.80
Carrot seed:	10ml	£7.90
Cedarwood:	10ml	£3.75
Chamomile Roman:	5ml	£14.00
Camomile German:	5ml	£25.00
Cinnamon:	10ml	£3.50
Citronella:	10ml	£3.75
Clary sage:	5ml	£5.00 – £7.00
Clove:	5ml	£3.75
Coriander:	5ml	£6.00 – £9.00
Cypress:	10ml	£6.00

Eucalyptus:	10ml	£3.50
Fennel:	10ml	£4.00
Frankincense:	5ml	£6.50
Geranium:	10ml	£5.50
Ginger:	10ml	£6.50
Grapefruit:	10ml	£4.00
Jasmine:	2ml	£20.00
Juniper:	10ml	£7.00
Lavender:	10ml	£4.00 – £7.00
Lemon:	10ml	£3.75
Lemongrass:	10ml	£3.75
Mandarin:	10ml	£5.50
Marjoram:	10ml	£5.00 – £10.00
Melissa:	10ml	£4.40
Melissa:	(true) 2ml	£25.00
Myrrh:	5ml	£4.00 – £10.00
Neroli:	2ml	£13.75 – £20.00
Niaouli:	10ml	£6.00
Orange:	10ml	£3.75
Palmarosa:	10ml	£5.00
Patchouli:	10ml	£4.00
Peppermint:	10ml	£3.75
Petitgrain:	10ml	£4.00
Pine:	10ml	£3.00 – £5.00
Rose:	2ml	From £11.00 absolute – £30 for rose otto
Rosemary:	10ml	£3.75
Rosewood:	10ml	£4.00
Sandalwood:	5ml	£4.00
Tangerine:	10ml	£5.50
Tea tree:	10ml	£4.00 – £8.00
Vetivert:	5ml	£4.00 – £6.00
Ylang-ylang:	10ml	£6.00

Apricot kernel:	100ml	£4.00
Avocado:	100ml	£6.00
Grapeseed:	100ml	£3.00
Jojoba:	100ml	£9.00
Peach kernel:	100ml	£8.00
Sweet almond:	100ml	£3.20
Wheatgerm:	100ml	£4.75

Prices may vary slightly from supplier to supplier depending on availability, harvests, weather and quality.

A STARTER'S KIT:
SELECTING OILS FOR
EVERYDAY USE

Faced with the choice of so many oils, it can be a daunting task for a newcomer to aromatherapy to select the ones they need. This chapter will recommend oils that you will find of maximum benefit and value for money and suggest how to use them to treat various common ailments.

A STARTER KIT

Deciding which oils to include in this section was no easy task as each oil has its own particular merit and healing ability. In the end, I opted for the following 12 oils to include in your bathroom cabinet for a variety of reasons:

- Their versatility – to allow maximum use and therefore value for money.

- Their therapeutic properties and potency to relieve common complaints on both the physical, mental and emotional level.

- Pure indulgence.

- Availability and low cost.

...pe you will find them of use and representative of all the ...est that the oils have to offer. You will be able to use them:

A) To prevent everyday disorders manifesting.

B) As natural alternatives to the synthetically made potions and pills on sale.

C) Simply for the experience.

This basic kit will work for: colds, coughs, headaches, hang-overs, sinusitis, insomnia, stomach upset, depression, sports injuries, stress and swelling.

NB. If you find after reading this chapter that your particular needs don't seem to have been covered with these 12 oils, for a complete list of all the oils and their uses see the appendices.

To find out what the various properties referred to in the list mean e.g. haemostatic = stems the flow of blood, turn to the appendices for a list of the meanings.

THE TWELVE OILS

1) Basil

2) Bergamot

3) Camomile

4) Eucalyptus

5) Juniper

6) Lavender

7) Lemon

8) Peppermint

9) Rosemary

10) Sandalwood

11) Tea tree

12) Ylang-ylang

1) BASIL (OCIMUM BASILICUM)

Origins:
  Bulgaria/USA/Madagascar, Seychelles/Asia/Europe

Plant part used:
  whole plant

Used for:
  mental fatigue, nerve tonic, bronchitis, migraine, gout, loss of concentration, colds, asthma, fainting, to regulate menstrual cycle, coughs, digestive disorders, vomiting, wasp and insect bites

Main constituents:
  borneone, camphor, cineol, eugenol, pinene, sylvestrene, methylchavicol, ocimene, linalol

Properties:
  analgesic, antidepressant, antiseptic, emmenagogue, expectorant, insecticide, tonic

Scent:
  herbaceous, clear, sweet

Method of extraction:
  distillation

Particularly good for:
   mental fatigue

Warning:
   if used to excess can be a depressant. It is emmenagogue so best to avoid in pregnancy.

In practice:
- A few drops on a tissue for mental fatigue, inhale when studying, in a meeting, before an exam or whenever concentration is flagging

- In a morning bath with bergamot to awaken, refresh and invigorate (6 to 8 drops, i.e. four of each oil)

- Use neat on a cotton bud on wasp stings

- A few drops on a wet flannel left on a radiator will purify the atmosphere, strengthen in the case of nervous or mental fatigue as well as help clear a cold in head or headache

2) BERGAMOT (CITRUS BERGAMIA)

Origins:
   Ivory Coast/Italy/Morocco/Guinea

Plant part used:
   peel of fruit

Used for:
   acne, skin problems, herpes, tension, depression, stress, fevers, cystitis, restore appetite

Main constituents:
   linalyl acetate, limonene, linalol, bergaptene, nerol, terpineol

Properties:
  antiseptic, antidepressant, antiviral, analgesic, antispasmodic, tonic

Scent:
  light, citrus, refreshing

Method of extraction:
  expression

Particularly good for:
  depression as it is uplifting, tonic, skin problems

Warning:
  avoid sunbathing or using a sunbed after use as it can cause problems of skin pigmentation

In practice:
- 6 drops in an aromatic bath to uplift and refresh in the morning

- In massage oil for depression

- A few drops on a wet flannel left on a radiator to awaken and clear the head in the morning

- Add a few drops to your skin toner for problem free skin

- A few drops on a gauze compress for acne sufferers. Add a few drops of oil to a bowl of warm water, soak the gauze in it, wring out and place over the face for few minutes every day until symptoms clear

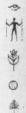

3) CAMOMILE (CHAMAMELUM NOBILE/ORMENSIS MULTICAULIS/MATRICARIA RECUTICA)

Origins:
England/France/Hungary/Egypt/Morocco/Bulgaria/
Yugoslavia

Plant part used:
flowers/leaves

Used for:
calming, inflammation, insomnia, menstrual problems, nerves, stress, anxiety, irritability, digestive/stomach disorders, sprains/swollen joints, allergies, skin problems, acne, psoriasis, eczema, headaches, migraine, eye problems

Main constituents:
bisabolol, chamazulene, esters, linalol, pinene, azulene, tigilic

Properties:
antiseptic, analgesic, antispasmodic, anti-inflammatory, emmenagogue, sedative, stomachic, vulnerary

Scent:
pungent, strong, herbaceous

Method of extraction:
distillation

Particularly good for:
calming, inflammation, stomach upset, eye problems like conjunctivitis (never put the oil directly into the eye as it will

sting,) use as an analgesic

Warning:
avoid in the early months of pregnancy

In practice:

- For conjunctivitis, apply with a cotton pad soaked in luke-warm water to which a few drops of the oil have been added, then the pad wrung out

- A few drops on a hot compress (a flannel or small towel which has been soaked in hot water then wrung out) can bring great relief to menstrual cramps, stomach ache or lower back pain

- 1 drop in a baby's or toddler's bath for overtiredness to help unwind or in skin lotion to soothe nappy rashes or skin

4) EUCALYPTUS (EUCALYPTUS GLOBULUS/CITRIODORA)

Origins:
China/Australia/Spain/Brazil/California

Plant part used:
leaves/twigs

Used for:
coughs, bronchitis, sore throat, sinusitis, rheumatism, skin infections, viral infections, migraine, herpes, mosquito repel-lent, strained muscles, urinary tract problems, cystitis

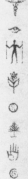

Main constituents:
    cineol, pinene, limonene, camphene, citronellal, fenchene, phellandrene

Properties:
    powerful antiseptic, anti-inflammatory, analgesic, antiviral, balsamic, decongestant, expectorant, antibacterial, diuretic, insecticide, antirheumatic

Scent:
    sweet, menthol

Method of extraction:
    steam distillation

Particularly good for:
    chest complaints, flu and colds viruses

Warning:
    avoid with homoeopathic remedies

In practice:
- In a steam inhalation for colds, catarrh, coughs and flu

- In massage for strained muscles or rheumatic complaints

- A few drops on a wet towel placed on the radiator will purify the air (as it is antiviral), plus give any sick room a fresh, clean smell

- As a mosquito repellent, add a few drops to your bath when abroad plus dilute four drops in some carrier oil and apply particularly around the ankles before going out in the evening

Origins:
Tyrol/India/North Africa/North America/North Asia/Europe

Plant part used:
berries

Used for:
liver problems, purification, detoxifying, acne, urinary infections, diuretic, obesity, appetite stimulant, period pains, eczema, psoriasis, ulcers, wounds, hangovers, rheumatism, cellulite, painful menstruation, sluggishness

Main constituents:
limonene, myrcene, pinene, borneol, terpineol, camphene, cadinene, sabinene

Properties:
diuretic, antiseptic, analgesic, antispasmodic, insecticide, stimulant, carminative

Scent:
clean, herbaceous

Particularly good for:
cleansing the system, hangovers, fluid retention, cellulite

Method of extraction:
steam distillation

Warning:
avoid if pregnant or suffering with kidney problems

In practice:
- 6 drops in an aromatic bath for water retention

- 3 drops of juniper/3 of bergamot in the bath to help clear the system and combat a hungover feeling

- For acne, add a few drops to your skincare products or add a few drops to a bowl of steaming water and use as a facial sauna

- For eczema, apply a few drops of juniper oil/a few drops of camomile diluted in carrier oil such as grapeseed to the afflicted limb

6) LAVENDER (LAVANDULA VERA/AUGUSTIFOLIUM/OFFICINALIS)

Origins:
France/Bulgaria/Yugoslavia/England/Tasmania

Plant part used:
flowering tops

Used for:
burns, skin infections, skincare, cuts, wounds, acne, eczema, dermatitis, flu, nausea, stress, headaches, asthma, rheumatism, arthritis, cystitis, high blood pressure, muscle spasm, arthritis, muscular aches and pains, sunburn, fainting, insomnia, respiratory problems, allergies

Main constituents:

acetate, cineol, caryophyllene, linalol, linalyl acetate, lavadulyl acetate, geraniol, borneol, limonene, pinene

Properties:

highly antiseptic, analgesic, antirheumatic, antiviral, antispasmodic, carminative, emmenagogue, sedative, antidepressant, decongestant, vulnerary

Scent:

clean, light, floral

Particularly good for:

stress, headaches, cuts, burns, warts

Method of extraction:

steam distillation

In practice:

- A few drops on the pillow to aid sleep

- In a massage (diluted in carrier oil) for stress or general aches and pains

- Neat on a cotton pad or cotton bud for cuts, burns, stings or bruises

- A few drops on a wet towel placed on a radiator to purify and scent a sick room (lavender smells wonderfully clean and will remove any cloying stuffy smell that can sometimes linger in a room where someone is unwell)

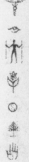

7) LEMON (CITRUS LIMONUM)

Origins:
Spain/Brazil/Israel/USA/Argentina

Plant part used:
fruit rind

Used for:
digestive problems, sore throat, a nervous tonic, skin problems, insect repellent, arthritis, lowers blood pressure, cardiac stimulant, liver purifier, colds, flu, sinusitis, gingivitis, nosebleeds, corns, warts and verrucas

Main constituents:
bergaptene, citral, camphene, limonene, pinene, linalol, cadinene, bisabolene, phellandrene

Properties:
highly antiseptic, tonic, astringent, antiacid, diuretic, bactericide, emollient, hypotensive, antirheumatic, laxative, haemostatic

Scent:
light, citrus, refreshing, sharp

Particularly good for:
skin problems (acne, greasy skin), tonic

Method of extraction:
expression

after use avoid sun or sunbeds for six to eight hours.
Can irritate sensitive skin

In practice:

- In a morning bath to refresh

- A few drops added to skincare products (cleanser, toner and moisturizer) will add a pleasant scent plus make them all more effective. Lemon is said to help prevent wrinkles and is anti-ageing

- A few drops in the final rinse water when washing hair for shine, scent and a clean healthy scalp

- Gargle a few drops in warm water (with 2 drops of sandalwood) for sore throats

8) PEPPERMINT (MENTHA PIPERASCENS)

Origins:
England/America/China/Europe

Plant part used:
whole plant

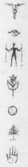

Used for:
nausea, flatulence, colic, indigestion, travel sickness, headaches, colds, flu, migraine, fevers, inflammation, arthritis, sinusitis, painful periods, mosquito repellent, asthma, bronchitis, fatigue, shock

Main constituents:
cineol, menthol, menthene, carvone, jasmone, carvacrol, limonene, phellandrene

PRINCIPLES OF AROMATHERAPY

Properties:
decongestant, antispasmodic, stimulating, analgesic, anaesthetic, antiseptic, carminative, hepatic

Scent:
minty, menthol, refreshing

Method of extraction:
steam distillation

Particularly good for:
headaches, travel sickness, colds and flu

Warning:
avoid use with homoeopathic remedies, also it can disturb sleep if used too near bedtime and can irritate the skin if used in too high a dosage

In practice:
- Put a few drops on a cold wrung out wet towel and use as a compress placed on the forehead. It is very effective for bringing relief for headaches

- Keep a bottle in the glove compartment of your car and put a few drops on a tissue to be inhaled by anyone suffering from travel sickness on car journeys. The scent will also help keep the driver alert

- A few drops in steam inhalation for colds and flu

Origins:
  Spain/Tunisia/Zimbabwe/France/Japan/Yugoslavia

Plant part used:
  flowers/leaves

Used for:
  headaches, muscular strains, sports injuries, sprains, fatigue, dandruff, alopecia, stimulant, liver decongestant, rheumatism, colds, improves circulation, intestinal upsets, fluid retention, coughs, chest congestion

Main constituents:
  camphor, cineol, camphene, bornyl acetate, borneol, pinene, cuminic, borneol

Properties:
  antiseptic, antibacterial, antifungal, diuretic, stimulating, antidepressant, antispasmodic, diuretic, emmenagogue, hypertensive, tonic, vulnerary

Scent:
  fresh, herbaceous, slightly menthol, piercing

Method of extraction:
  steam distillation

Particularly good for:
  sprains, sports injuries, strained muscles, use as a tonic

Warning:
avoid in pregnancy or if you have epilepsy

In practice:
- In massage, use a few drops diluted in carrier oil for strained or aching muscles and rheumatism

- 4–6 drops on a cold compress placed on a sprain can relieve the pain and bring down swelling

- A few drops added to hair products to prevent and combat dandruff

- 6 drops in the bath or in massage oil for fluid retention

- A few drops in a steam inhalation for colds and flu symptoms

10) SANDALWOOD (SANTALUM ALBUM)

Origins:
East India/Indonesia

Plant part used:
wood

Used for:
acne, cystitis, sunstroke, sore throats, bronchitis, laryngitis, urinary tract problems, fluid retention, skin problems, acne, psoriasis, eczema, sores, chapped or dry skin, skincare, stress

Main constituents:
santalol, furfurol, santalene, fusanol

Properties:
 antiseptic, diuretic, antispasmodic, expectorant, sedative, aphrodisiac, diuretic

Scent:
 gentle, warm, woody

Particularly good for:
 skin problems, sore throats, urinary tract complaints

Method of extraction:
 distillation

In practice:

- Added to skin products will aid their effectiveness

- A few drops added to warm water then gargled will help relief for sore throats

- In a carrier oil for massage for relaxation

- To help eczema, put 4 drops in carrier oil and apply to the afflicted area (can be used in combination with juniper, camomile or lavender for this)

- A few drops in the bath or in massage oil for use as an aphrodisiac

11) TEA TREE/TI-TREE (MELALEUCA ALTERNIFOLIA)

Origins:
 Australia/Tasmania

Plant part used:
 leaves/twigs

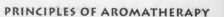

Used for:
fungal infections, viral and bacterial infections, colds, flu, cold sores, acne, cystitis, candida, burns, athlete's foot, insect repellent, cuts, cold sores, stings, sore throats, sinusitis, chest problems, dandruff, verrucas and warts, to strengthen the immune system to fight infection

Main constituents:
cineol, cymene, pinene, terpineol, terpinene

Properties:
powerful antiseptic, antifungal, antibiotic, antiviral, expectorant, insecticide

Scent:
disinfectant, medicinal

Particularly good for:
cuts, cold sores, genital infections

Method of extraction:
steam distillation

In practice:
- For cuts, burns and stings use neat with a cotton bud or pad

- For colds, flu and coughs, use a few drops in a steam inhalation. Although an extremely potent oil for fighting infection, it is one of the gentlest oils to inhale

- 6 drops in the bath for urinary tract problems or a few drops in a douche

- Neat on a cotton bud for cold sores
- 4 drops in a warm foot bath for athlete's foot, then apply carrier oil containing a few drops of tea tree

12) YLANG-YLANG (CANANGA ODORATA)

Origins:
Comora Islands/Indonesia/Phillipines/Seychelles

Plant part used:
flowers

Used for:
anxiety, lowers high blood pressure, depression, aphrodisiac, regulates and calms the heart, skincare, sexual problems (frigidity, impotence)

Main constituents:
benzyl acetate, geraniol, linalol, pinene, benzoic, farnesol, eugenol, cadinene

Properties:
aphrodisiac, antiseptic, antidepressant, hypotensive, sedative

Scent:
floral, heady

Particularly good for:
relaxation, its scent and feelgood factor

Method of extraction:
steam distillation

In practice:

- 6 drops in the bath for pure indulgence, relaxation and heady scent

- For an effective aphrodisiac, 3 drops of ylang-ylang with 3 drops of sandalwood diluted in a massage oil

- Add a few drops to your skincare products for scent and blooming, healthy skin

- A few drops on a tissue will help anyone who suffers from nerves or heart palpitations

- 6 drops diluted in massage oil to help reduce stress and lower blood pressure

- For perfume, 4 drops on a wet towel placed on the radiator

The oils can also be used in combination. For example:

3

FOR COLDS AND FLU
Eucalyptus/rosemary
Eucalyptus/tea tree
Eucalyptus/peppermint

FOR HEADACHES
Lavender/camomile
Lavender/peppermint

FOR MENTAL FATIGUE
Basil/peppermint
Rosemary/bergamot

FOR ECZEMA
Lavender/camomile
Lavender/juniper

FOR STRESS
Lavender/camomile
Lavender/ylang-ylang
Sandalwood/lavender

DETOXIFYING/HANGOVERS/CELLULITE
Juniper/rosemary

SKINCARE
Lemon/lavender
Camomile/sandalwood
Bergamot/sandalwood

FOR WOUNDS
Camomile/lavender
Tea tree/lavender

CYSTITIS
Sandalwood/lavender
Tea tree/sandalwood

REFRESHING
Lemon/basil
Bergamot/rosemary

SORE THROATS
Sandalwood/lemon
Sandalwood/teatree

FOR PURIFYING SICK ROOM
Eucalyptus/peppermint
Lavender/lemon

6

AROMATHERAPY
FOR STRESS RELIEF

THE NEED

As we draw near to the end of the twentieth century, stress is an unavoidable part of many people's lives. As life becomes increasingly fraught – inner cites with their rising crime rates, overcrowding, escalating prices – it's no wonder the general public experience more and more stress.

As the problem grows so does the need to find a way to alleviate it and yet every day, people soldier on against setbacks and frustrations which can vary from the minor such as traffic or public transport to the major such as redundancy or divorce. We put all sorts of worries, financial, emotional and physical, to the back of our minds as we go about our daily lives.

In the past, people were encouraged to keep a stiff upper lip, to bury anxieties and just get on with the necessary hurly-burly of survival; many are still tempted to take this road. However, our systems do need rejuvenating, recharging and revitalizing. Regularly, we take our cars in for a service but how many people treat their bodies with the same consideration? It is important to give the body a chance to unwind, be realigned, pampered, soothed, re-energized.

Aromatherapy is one of the most effective methods of doing

this. Also by treating the early unease of stress helps prevent later physical symptoms of disease, which could have more serious implications, from manifesting.

In the last decade, a remarkable swing has taken place regarding the popularity of healthy alternatives. Responding to this growing need, health centres, clinics and practitioners are springing up all over the country. Interest has grown in therapies such as aromatherapy. Once it was viewed as slightly cranky or indulgent, but now it has a respected place with those involved in healthcare. The media has also recognized and addressed the need for relaxation and the benefits of treatments such as aromatherapy in many of its magazines and journals.

WHAT CAUSES STRESS?

The list is long and probably familiar:

EMOTIONAL STRESS

- Death of loved ones

- Divorce (separation), loss

- Personal relationships

- Children

PHYSICAL STRESS

- Illness

- Being in a hurry

- Bad diet: fast foods

- Physical stresses: driving, lifting, standing all day, typing all day, extremes of temperature and temperature changes

- Extremes of exercise, excessive or none
- Lack of exercise
- Moving house
- A new baby
- Overworking
- Holidays/Christmas
- A fast lifestyle which ignores the needs of the mind and body

ENVIRONMENTAL STRESS

- Public transport
- Inadequate office facilities: too cramped, bad lighting, bad chairs resulting in aches and bad posture
- Noise levels
- Traffic
- Crowded public facilities

MENTAL STRESS

- Performance at work, pressure to succeed
- Tests, exams
- Finances
- Frustration at work, job dissatisfaction
- Retirement
- Job uncertainty
- Redundancy
- Enforced change

ISN'T IT ENOUGH JUST TO RELAX AT HOME?

In theory yes but in practice no, because quite simply many people don't truly relax and unwind during their time off. Living as we do in a fast-moving society with one in three marriages ending in divorce, threat of redundancies, job uncertainty, it is no wonder that to many people, the art of relaxation is lost. Emotional worries result in sleepless nights, mental worries manifest as irritation, concern about children and their education which results in anxiety.

Many people's way of relaxing at home is to switch off with a gin and tonic or a glass of wine and while there is nothing wrong with this in moderation, it doesn't deal with any stress, alleviate the root of it or replenish the system. Others smoke when under stress, overeat or take drugs, all of which can at worst become a dependency, at the least take their toll in taxing the system rather than relaxing it.

If people truly knew how to cope with stress, the doctors wouldn't be writing out endless prescriptions for tranquillizers and antidepressants.

For the majority of us, we need to find a healthy alternative which enables us to let go and shut off from everyday concerns without resorting to quick fixes whose benefits in the long run are questionable.

CAN STRESS BE DANGEROUS?

Stress can be draining in the short-term and serious to health if ignored in the long-term. If left untreated, stress can develop from a minor disorder into major illness. Medical research is finding many major illnesses such as cancer and heart failure are linked to stress. Yet if symptoms are treated and stress released as soon as it manifests, it reduces the chances of it developing into anything more serious.

WHAT ARE THE SYMPTOMS OF STRESS?

There are many symptoms and manifestations of stress. It affects people to varying degrees. Stressful situations can effect a person either physically, mentally or emotionally depending on their particular way of dealing with life. For example, a person may get a bill that he cannot meet, he may think he's unaffected but nevertheless, the stress is stored physically in his shoulders resulting in tense muscles or a headache. Another person may worry about the bills but in this case, it may cause irritability and lack of sleep.

Another example is a driver who has a near miss on the road; relieved she escaped, she breathes a sigh of relief and continues on her way. Only most likely, she won't have escaped completely unblemished. The stress of the incident will be stored somewhere in the body, perhaps in the neck from when she tensed up, perhaps mentally so as she continues her journey, she is jumpy and nervous about traffic.

Same situation, different responses, all resulting in a type of stress which is so often left untreated as we move on to the next day or hurdle.

Here's a list of some of the ways stress can manifest:

Physically:
migraine; headaches; insomnia; tense, strained muscles; ulcers; bloating; loss of appetite; exhaustion; tight stomach; shallow breathing; high blood pressure; muscle tension; teeth grinding during sleep; increased heart rate; extra adrenalin; increased perspiration; weakened immune system; tendency to come down with every virus in the work place; feeling run

down; irritable bowel syndrome; nerves; excessive cravings for
alcohol; caffeine; tobacco; sugar; skin rashes.

Mentally:

lack of concentration; irritation; mental fatigue; anxiety; anger; apathy; lack of sex drive; fear; burn out; forgetfulness.

Emotionally:

mood swings; tearfulness; depression; lack of confidence; grief.

HOW CAN I USE AROMATHERAPY TO RELIEVE STRESS?

1) First admit that you suffer from stress.

It is said that the first step to finding your way is to admit that you're lost. In the same way, the first step to relaxation is to acknowledge that you're under stress – so if you suffer from any of the symptoms above then you'd probably benefit from all that aromatherapy has to offer in the way of stress relief.

2) Book regular sessions with an aromatherapist.

Depending on how demanding your work schedule is, try to book sessions every two weeks, failing that every four weeks. Make it a priority, a necessary part of your working life. It will certainly help improve your performance. Under stress, people's decision-making can become clouded, their judgement impaired. When relaxed, body and mind function better.

A practitioner, as well as giving you an aromatherapy massage, will also look at your lifestyle and diet, suggest oils for home use and ways that you can practically reduce the stress levels in your life.

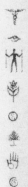

3) If you cannot afford either the time or the money for treatments with a practitioner, you can still gain from aromatherapy by using some of the oils at home.

   The list below shows which oils can be used to alleviate which symptom of stress.

   - The oils can be used either for massage or in an aromatic bath as described in Chapter 3.
   - The oils can be used either on their own or in combination with one or two of the other oils also listed for a particular condition. For example for a headache you could use just 6 drops of lavender in a bath or massage or you could combine 2 drops of lavender with 2 drops of marjoram and 2 drops of camomile.

FOR PHYSICAL SYMPTOMS

Migraine:
   peppermint, lavender, camomile

Skin rashes:
   camomile, lavender, benzoin

Headaches:
   lavender, peppermint, basil, marjoram, eucalyptus

Insomnia:
   marjoram, camomile, lavender, neroli

Tense, strained muscles:
   lavender, rosemary, juniper, ginger

Ulcers:
   camomile, lavender, garlic

Bloating:
juniper, clary sage, fennel, geranium

Loss of appetite:
cinnamon, fennel, camomile, bergamot, cardamom

Exhaustion:
rosemary, black pepper, lemon, bergamot, peppermint

Tight stomach:
lavender, camomile, sandalwood, clary sage

Shallow breathing:
eucalyptus, basil, benzoin, melissa, marjoram

High blood pressure:
lavender, marjoram, ylang-ylang, camomile, neroli, rose

Muscle tension:
lavender, rosemary, clary sage, camomile

Teeth grinding during sleep:
marjoram, melissa, neroli

Increased heart rate:
ylang-ylang, camomile, neroli, lavender

Increased adrenalin:
lavender, marjoram, camomile

Weakened immune system, tendency to come down with every virus in the work place:
niaouli

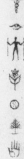

Feeling run down:
   rosemary, eucalyptus, ginger, cinnamon, lemon

Irritable bowel syndrome:
   rosemary, ginger, rose, lemongrass, orange

Nerves:
   lemon, neroli, camomile, patchouli, sandalwood, benzoin, tangerine

FOR MENTAL SYMPTOMS

Lack of concentration:
   basil, peppermint

Irritation:
   sandalwood, camomile, lavender, neroli

Mental fatigue:
   basil, peppermint, bergamot

Anxiety:
   melissa, clary sage, rosewood, neroli, patchouli

Anger:
   sandalwood, rosewood, neroli

Apathy:
   jasmine, black pepper, lemon

Lack of sex drive:
   ylang-ylang, sandalwood, clary sage, rose, ginger

Fear:
melissa, camomile

Burn-out:
lavender, bergamot, rosemary

Forgetfulness:
rosewood, sandalwood, basil

FOR EMOTIONAL SYMPTOMS

Mood swings:
geranium, sandalwood

Tearfulness:
jasmine

Depression:
jasmine, bergamot, clary sage, rose, sandalwood

Lack of confidence:
jasmine, ylang-ylang

Grief:
rose, rosewood, melissa, lavender

WHAT ARE THE BENEFITS OF AROMATHERAPY FOR STRESS?

PHYSICAL

Lower blood pressure

Better circulation

Relaxed muscles

MENTAL

Greater tolerance of people and situations

Increased appreciation of life

EMOTIONAL

A feeling of well-being

Emotional stability

Although we often blame circumstances, situations or other people for problems, actually, a good or bad experience is determined by state of mind. It is our response or reaction to a particular event or experience that leaves a memory rather than simply what's happening on the outside. We experience life on the inside. Hence peace of mind is very important. You can be in the most glorious of situations – on a beach in the Caribbean – and feeling lousy and uptight. You can be in the rain in the rush hour and feel you're in heaven because you're feeling good inside.

If you're feeling relaxed and mellow inwardly, an irritable colleague at work or family member at home can be dealt with in a reasonable manner. However if uptight and exhausted, the slightest thing can be the last straw and leave us feeling we can't cope another moment.

One of the wonderful things about aromatherapy is its ability to work on three levels. It relaxes the body, it can help the most active mind wind down and it can uplift someone feeling low. Achieving a more tranquil state of mind will help you overcome the everyday demands of life.

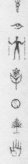

AROMATHERAPY AS AN AID TO WEIGHT LOSS

adly, there is no miracle oil to help you lose weight. The only lasting way is through cutting down what you eat and a sensible program of diet and exercise. However, although there is no fast solution to shedding the pounds, aromatherapy still has much to offer anyone who is concerned about their weight as the essential oils can be used in several ways as part of a weight loss regime.

GETTING THE RIGHT ATTITUDE

The first step to losing weight is actually nothing to do with diet or exercise. Like any lifestyle change, it has to come from the inside, from a desire to change the state of things. Sadly this often comes about when people have hit rock bottom. As many people turn to food when they are depressed, to comfort eat as if the food can fill an emptiness, it can start a cycle that can be hard to break, a vicious circle where they feel depressed, so eat, then feel stressed and low as they have broken the regime.

Aromatherapy can help. The uplifting oils can alleviate the feeling of being low and break the chain of negative feelings leading to overeating and lack of self worth. Sometimes a dieter needs something to lift them out of the circle, inspiration to feel good about themselves so that they want to make an effort.

Using the essential oils to relieve stress and build a sense of well-being can be the first step to making a positive effort in combating a weight problem. Your body gets the message that it matters. If you are feeling healthy and vital it is always easier to make the choices that are best for you.

The following oils can be used in the bath or in a massage:

Bergamot – uplifting, good for depression

Jasmine – gives a sense of inner beauty and inner joy

Rose – evokes a sense of the feminine and of lightness which is important as if even only slightly overweight, it is easy to think of yourself as 'a lump'

Ylang-ylang – gives a mellow feeling and sense of well-being and lightness

Rosewood – calming and uplifting

Geranium – helps restore balance. Often when embarking on a diet, people are attracted by extremes. They want fast results and will do mad diets to get results. Geranium can help restore balance both to mind and body

The first step to looking good on the outside is to feel good on the inside. These oils will all enhance this sense of self worth and help bring out a feeling of new determination.

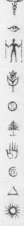

PAMPERING AS
AN ALTERNATIVE TO EATING

There's no doubting the fact that if you are on a diet you are having to make some sacrifices. Even though these days, all the nutritionists advise a sensible diet with no extremes and allowing for a little of what you fancy, it can still feel as if it's all work and no play. No indulgence in favourite foods, no comfort eating or little titbits to reward hard work or a job well done. This is where aromatherapy comes in.

Book yourself the treat of a body massage or aromatherapy facial as a healthy alternative to food. Allow yourself an indulgence that is both luxurious but can also help your weight loss. Tell the practitioner that you are on a diet and she can put oils in that can help if you have any particular stubborn areas or problems such as water retention or cellulite. Then lie back and enjoy someone else doing the work. The fact that you are spending some time on yourself will also help reinforce the message that you matter, you care about your body. This will build your sense of self worth, an attitude that does help in the dieting process.

DIURETIC AND DETOXIFYING OILS

Juniper/rosemary/fennel are all excellent for a system that retains water or is congested and in need of a clear-out. The reason this happens can be due to several causes:

1) Unhealthy diet and lifestyle

2) The beginning of the menstrual cycle or the beginning of the menopause

3) Allergies

4) Stress

The diuretics and detoxifying oils are good when the system has become congested and isn't working to maximum efficiency due to an unhealthy diet and lifestyle over a prolonged period of time.

Excess sugar, alcohol, coffee and fast foods all contribute to slowing down the system. The digestion has to fight to keep up with foods that are bulky but low in nutrition, in the case of excess alcohol, the liver is particularly affected. As the system grows acidic, it holds on to fluid to try and dilute this and so the best advice for anyone suffering from water retention due to unhealthy diet is to drink more water.

This may seem contradictory and many people with the condition think if they drink more water, they'll retain it and so settle for diuretic tablets instead. In fact, the more water you drink, the better your whole system can work. The more water you drink, the faster the toxicity can be dealt with and eliminated. Once excess toxicity has been dealt with, the system no longer needs to retain water as the system is clear. Many overweight people don't drink enough so inhibiting the body's natural elimination process.

If embarking on a healthy restart, the above oils can be used to give the whole system a bit of stimulation to work efficiently.

PREMENSTRUAL TENSION

Just before a period, many women retain a little more water than normal but it is usually eliminated straight after the period. The diuretic oils could be used in massage or in a bath to help alleviate the symptoms before the period starts.

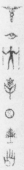

ALLERGY

Some people retain water because of an allergy to something they are eating. The most common allergies have been found to be wheat, coffee and dairy products. If you suspect that you are allergic to something, a good nutritionist will be able to help you in pinpointing what exactly it is. Many digestive complaints are also tied in with allergies and many sufferers have reported that once they have found out what their particular allergy is and eliminated it from their diet, all sorts of conditions have improved from irritable bowel syndrome to skin complaints to irritability and insomnia. Effortless weight loss is often reported.

STRESS

Stress can inhibit all of the body's major functions. It can diminish the circulation and lymph drainage. The best solution is regular deep relaxing massage using any of the oils good for unwinding such as lavender, marjoram, rosewood, sandalwood, neroli.

LYMPH DRAINAGE

Amongst the functions of the lymphatic system are:

the drainage of fluids

the drainage and elimination of toxic wastes

the absorption of fat into the intestines

It is important that this system is working efficiently. If it is clogged, it can result in sluggishness, bloating, fatigue, water retention and cellulite. Lymph drainage is a particular system of massage known to many aromatherapists and is becoming increasingly popular as it can relieve all these symptoms and help the lymph system work to maximum efficiency. Following the lines of the lymph in the body, i.e. from the hands to the armpits and the ankles to the groin and up to the collarbone, the practitioner will gently massage in oils that will help. For example:

Fennel – cleansing and diuretic.

Juniper – detoxifying, diuretic, good for overloaded liver.

Black pepper – stimulating.

Rosemary – cleansing, tonic, stimulating.

Geranium – balancing, diuretic.

Cypress – good for circulation.

If the lymph is working properly, those stubborn pounds will come off all the more easily.

At home, you can make use of these oils in the bath and do skin brushing daily. This is the vigorous brushing with swift strong movements along the lines of the lymph.

WEIGHT ASSOCIATED PROBLEMS

IRRITABLE BOWEL SYNDROME

Certain oils will aid the digestive system and help regulate the bowels. It isn't enough however just to use the oils. If you suffer from this condition, the best remedy is through changing your diet and advice from a nutritionist would be helpful. However, once a program has been embarked on, the oils could be used in conjunction to help normalize the system.

CONSTIPATION

As with irritable bowel syndrome, there is a reason that some people suffer from constipation. It is best remedied with:

A) Increasing the intake of water.

B) Carefully looking at the diet to see if there is an excess of foods that are causing the complaint. A change of diet to include more fibre, plenty of fresh vegetables and fruits and less red meat is usually recommended.

C) Using the oils in massage or aromatic baths to stimulate the bowels back into regular elimination. Oils that are good for constipation include: fennel, black pepper, marjoram, ginger, rosemary.

D) Looking at the lifestyle and perhaps introducing some exercise if it has been lacking all together.

CELLULITE

These are the fat deposits usually found around the hips, thighs buttocks and sometimes the upper arms and stomach. It has an uneven porridge-like appearance, like orange peel if squeezed. Although sometimes it is hereditary, the main causes are:

hormonal changes

bad circulation

smoking

bad diet

sugar

alcohol

lack of exercise

Although aromatherapy can help, as with all the weight related conditions, change has to come in all aspects of the lifestyle:

1) Diet: eat plenty of raw vegetables and fruit.

2) Regular exercise.

3) Skin brushing (as for lymph drainage).

4) Avoid sugar, coffee, alcohol, tobacco.

5) Drink 6 to 8 glasses of water a day.

6) Book regular sessions with an aromatherapist.

7) Take daily aromatic baths.

8) Make up your own blend for cellulite and apply nightly before sleep. The oils to use are three of any of the following: cypress, rosemary, fennel, black pepper, lemon, juniper, geranium or cedarwood diluted in a base oil. Use 10 drops to 20 ml of base oil.

9) Once a week, apply a hot compress which has been soaked in the oils mentioned above to the area where the cellulite is: then wrap the area in hot towels to help penetrate the skin and intensify the detoxification process.

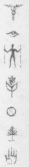

Cellulite doesn't appear in a week and certainly won't disappear overnight but the above steps will certainly help and you should see a notable difference in about six weeks. In order to remove it completely, you will have to practise these steps as part of your lifestyle.

STRETCH MARKS

Some people say that once the stretch marks have arrived, it is very difficult to get rid of them although they do fade with time. In this case, all that can be done is to improve the condition and tone of the skin.

With this is mind, prevention is the next best step. If you are embarking on a weight loss program and intend to lose a lot of weight, then begin using the oils to help prevent stretch marks at the beginning. Don't wait until the weight has gone.

The oils for this condition are mandarin, tangerine and neroli. Apply them nightly diluted in body lotion or oil.

HIGH BLOOD PRESSURE

Often people who are very overweight suffer from high blood pressure. As it puts strain on the heart and in extreme cases can lead to heart failure and kidney failure, it is obviously not a condition that should be overlooked or taken lightly. Measures should be taken to reduce stress, improve the diet and general lifestyle and an appointment with a doctor or nutritionist would be advisable to see exactly what steps should be taken.

Oils that can help reduce hypertension include: marjoram, clary sage, lavender, ylang-ylang. These can be used in the bath as well as in massage.

8

AROMATHERAPY AS A BEAUTY AID

With the choice of products available these days, the consumer can end up spending a fortune on beauty products and never be really sure whether what they're paying for is the product, the packaging or its advertising.

I have found that the oils mentioned in this chapter for beauty products are the most effective I've ever come across, particularly for the skin. The properties of the essential oils make both potent and natural ingredients for a whole range of products which won't break the bank, really do bring about positive results in all areas of beauty treatments, plus they soothe away any underlying tension and stress at the same time.

It must be said though, before I go into which oils are useful for the different skin types, that although you can apply no end of products and potions, the best results will come about if you combine the use of the essential oils with a healthy lifestyle paying particular attention to diet.

What we take into our bodies reflects very clearly in the condition of the skin. A badly balanced diet can result in spots and an oily complexion. Excess caffeine, alcohol and smoking can all contribute to a prematurely aged skin, at the least to a dry skin.

With skincare, all the following factors should be looked at and improved where possible:

Diet – avoid excess of over-refined foods, sugar and alcohol

Stress

Lack of exercise

Lack of sleep

Illness

Not drinking enough water

Ineffective skincare

Over exposure to the sun and elements with inadequate protection

ESSENTIAL OILS AS PART OF A BEAUTY ROUTINE

You can choose any of three ways of using the essential oils as part of your beauty routine:

A) Add them to products you already use to enhance and boost their effectiveness.

B) Buy readymade aromatherapy products from health shops and suppliers listed at the back of this book.

C) Make up your own.

Although most people would be interested in using homemade products made with the essential oils, many can't be bothered with having to actually mix the bases and prepare toners, shampoos, creams and moisturizers from scratch.

This needn't be a problem. Many suppliers and health shops sell neutral bases that have no chemical additives or scent to which you can add the essential oils of your choice.

New Seasons (whose address is given in the appendices) supplies everything you might need to make your own personalized toiletries. Their products range from toners (rosewater, witchhazel) to moisturizers, shampoos, hand cream and bath foam bases. They also sell the full range of different carrier oils (avocado, grapeseed, almond, peach kernel, jojoba, to name but a few).

Once you have your neutral base, you can experiment until you find the essential oils that fit your preferences and needs exactly.

In general you should add:

For the face: 3% essential oil to 97% base

For the body: 5% essential oil to 95% base

ESSENTIAL OILS AND THE SKIN

One of the things that makes the oils so effective in skincare is their ability to penetrate right to the bottom layer.

The skin is made up of three layers:

- The subcutaneous – this is the bottom layer and contains muscles and fatty tissue.

- The dermis – this is where the blood and lymph vessels, sensory nerves, hair follicles, sebaceous and sweat glands are located.

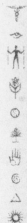

(The sweat glands produce perspiration which escapes through the pores of the skin. If these pores are blocked, spots and blackheads can result. The sebaceous glands produce the sebum which lubricates the skin, seals moisture into the cells and preserves the elasticity of the skin.)

Whether these glands are working effectively determines whether skin is dry, greasy or normal.

- The epidermis – the top layer which is made up primarily of dead cells. The cells in the skin are constantly renewing themselves. Cells made in the dermis travel to the top. (This is the process that slows down with age.)

Many products on the market today claim to be able to penetrate all three layers of the skin but in fact very few actually go right down to the subcutaneous layer.

The marvellous thing about the oils is that because of their molecular makeup, they can actually penetrate the skin's surface right down to the deepest layer and start improving all types of skin from within.

The skin can be fed, regenerated, stimulated, rebalanced or nourished depending on the individual's need. The natural antiseptic properties of the oils keep it clean and bacteria free.

DRY SKIN

The cause:

Dry skin comes about because the sebaceous glands are underactive and unable to produce the oil needed to prevent the skin losing moisture.

The solution:

What is needed are oils that will encourage the glands to

function normally again as well as moisturizing and nourish-
ing the skin.

Avoid:
 sun, sunbeds, alcohol, overheated houses.

Oils for dry skin:
 Geranium, rose, sandalwood, neroli, patchouli, ylang -ylang,
camomile.

Toner:
 Camomile, rosewater or rosehip toner.

Base oils:
> jojoba – leaves a satiny feeling.
>
> avocado – rich.
>
> sweet almond – easily absorbed.
>
> hazelnut – rich in vitmain E.

Add 10 per cent of wheatgerm oil to any of these mixtures to
help preserve it.

Weekly mask:
 A cup of oatmeal, spoon of almond oil, water, 4 drops of
essential oil. Mix, apply to the face and leave for ten minutes.

GREASY SKIN

Cause:
 In the case of oily skin, the sebaceous glands are overactive
and produce excess oil.

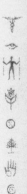

Solution:

What is needed are oils to redress the imbalance and aid the glands in working normally. It is important to keep the skin clean so that the pores don't get clogged with dust, makeup or debris. The antiseptic properties in oils help keep infection in check so helping to prevent spots and pimples.

It is also important to keep the skin lubricated by applying oil. Many people with greasy skin try to get their skin as dry as possible and try to remove all traces of oiliness. This starts a vicious circle as the sebaceous glands will only try and produce more oil to replace what is being removed or lost. The solution is to rebalance the glands, get to the root and keep the skin bacteria-free.

Avoid:

Coffee, sugar, fatty foods, spicy foods, sugar.

Toner:

Orange water or witchhazel (good decongestant).

Base oils:

People with oily skin prefer the lighter base oils that are more easily absorbed.

Grapeseed – very light.

Apricot, peach kernel – both are easily absorbed.

Oils for greasy skin:

Lemon, bergamot, juniper, geranium, sandalwood, neroli, lavender, tea tree. Lavender in particular will help if there is any scarring on the face as it will speed up the healing process.

Steaming the skin is good to keep pores clear. Add a few drops of juniper, lemon or lavender to a bowl of boiling water, cover your head with a towel and immerse the face in the steam, coming up for air when you need. Splash the skin afterwards to close the pores.

A hot compress could also be used. Take a clean flannel which has been soaked in hot water to which a few drops of any of the above essential oils has been added. Place the hot flannel over the face for a few minutes. Again afterwards, splash the skin with cold water to close the pores.

ACNE

Acne is also caused by overactive sebaceous glands. The oil build-up can cause blackheads, dandruff or eczema if not treated. The treatment of acne by the essential oils in combination with a healthy diet is very effective and any sufferer should see results within a month. All the recommendations given above will beneficial for anyone with acne.

AGEING SKIN

The cause:

The simple fact of growing old and the various elements encountered along the way leave their mark, from weather to the up and downs of life, they all take their toll on even the most well cared for skin.

Apart from that, it takes 120 days for new cells in the dermis to get to the surface and die. This process slows down with age and the surface cells are not replaced so frequently. This can result in a skin that can look weary and a little dull. The elastin and network of collagen in the dermis also slow down and lose their elasticity and as a result the skin loses its firmness and suppleness.

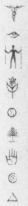

The solution:

Regular skincare is essential as you get older and although you can't halt the ageing process, you can certainly slow it down for a while. Exfoliation should be an important part of your program as this helps to remove the dead cells from the surface. Using essential oils to help stimulate new growth should be the next step and these oils can be added at all stages of the cleansing routine to cleansers, toners, and moisturizers. Don't forget the neck.

Avoid:

As with dry skin – sun, excess caffeine, alcohol, smoking, over-refined foods, stress.

Base oils:

People with older skins often want an oil or moisturizers that are a little heavier. Avocado, sesame, jojoba could all be used but if you find them too rich add a percentage of the lighter ones such as apricot or peach kernel. Again wheatgerm oil can be added to any mix to help preserve it.

Oils for an ageing skin:

Rose, frankincense, neroli, myrrh, lemon, patchouli, sandal-wood, carrot.

NORMAL SKIN

Cause:

Everything is working well, a good normal skin is either hereditary or due to good diet, good health and good care – though very few people have a completely normal skin. It usually tends to be on the dry side, on the oily side or even a combination. It is so important to look after the skin, no matter what age or condition. As with all aspects of aromatherapy, prevention is its main strength and the earlier you start treating your skin with such excellent products, the longer you can keep your skin looking good and glowing with health.

Solution:

Thorough skincare and regular use of the essential oils.

Base oils:

You can choose whichever you prefer although most people tend to like the lighter oils such as peach and apricot kernel.

Essential oils for normal skin:

Rose, lavender, lemon, neroli, bergamot, sandalwood, petit-grain, patchouli, rosewood, ylang-ylang

AN AROMATIC FACIAL ROUTINE:

Examples

DAILY:

Cleanse with cleanser containing any combination of essential oils for the skin, for example:

bergamot and sandalwood

geranium and lemon

lavender and camomile

Tone with witchhazel/orange flower water or rosewater to which has been added:

lemon and lavender

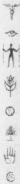

petitgrain and bergamot

lime and cedarwood

rosewood and rose

lemon and lime

Moisturize with a neutral base moisturizer to which has been added:

neroli, frankincense and rose

rose and lavender

ylang-ylang, lemon and sandalwood

jasmine and patchouli

myrrh and lemon

geranium, lemon, rosewood

WEEKLY:

Use a hot compress (clean flannel soaked in water to which a few drops of the oils have been added). You could use:

lavender

rose

geranium and sandalwood

frankincense and lemon

Leave the flannel on the skin for five minutes, then splash the skin with cold water to close the pores.

Eye mask:

to soothe tired or puffy eyes. Boil up a camomile tea bag, let the water cool slightly, add a drop of lavender or camomile oil. Squeeze excess water out of the bag and place on the eyes for a few minutes. The sensation is wonderfully soothing.

MONTHLY:

Exfoliate:

to help remove dead cells from the surface of the skin. Either buy an exfoliator to which you can add your essential oils or make one from one cup of oatmeal (either fine or coarse) depending on what you want, one teaspoon of clear honey, half a cup of ground almonds. Mix together. Add 6 drops of oil. Apply to the face. For this you could use geranium, sandalwood or bergamot

FACE MASK

Buy a clay mask and add a few drops of essential oil to it or pulp some fresh fruit such as apricots, peaches or even apples.

Some people like to add an egg or a teaspoonful of honey as these give the homemade masks more substance. Blend in the blender, add a few drops of essential oil and apply to the face for 10 minutes. (These fruit masks are good for the skin but tend to be a bit messy as they run, so make sure your hair is covered if you don't want to have to wash it afterwards!) Rose, sandalwood, lavender, ylang-ylang, rosewood or patchouli would all make good additions to any face mask.

EYE MASK

Can reduce puffiness after a late night or refresh eyes before an evening out after a long day's work in smokey conditions.

Camomile tea bags make the best eye masks as they are safe and non irritating. Simply boil up water and add to a cup

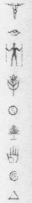

containing the tea bags as you would to make tea. Add a drop of essential oil to the liquid, neroli, camomile or lavender would do. Make sure the oil is well mixed in the water and soaked into the bag. Squeeze out the bag and place it on the eyes for a few minutes.

FOR BATHTIME

You can use the oils in several ways at bathtime.

1) Add 6 to 8 drops to the water swishing it around well.

2) Add the drops to a base oil which you apply before you get in the bath. This helps the oil absorb into the skin as the heat of the water will help the oils penetrate.

3) Add them to readymade bases, i.e. bath oils or bubble baths and foams.

4) Add the essential oils to your after bath lotion and apply all over.

The oils:

the following are so fragrant that they can be enough if used singularly to make bathtime a fragrant and relaxing experience:

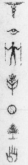

rose

jasmine

ylang-ylang

neroli

orange

bergamot

rosewood

geranium

sandalwood

patchouli

They could also be used in combination, for example:

For men:
  lime, lavender, cedarwood, bergamot, sandalwood

For women:
  lemon, ylang-ylang

Refreshing:
  rosemary, lemon,

Relaxing:
  lavender, rose

Exotic:
  Ylang-ylang, patchouli

Soothing:
  neroli, rosewood

Uplifting:
  jasmine, lemon

When adding to any lotion, 5 per cent essential oil to 95 per cent lotion or oil will be sufficient for the body. Use less if you're going to use this lotion on the skin on your face.

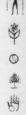

HANDS AND FEET

Add essential oils to an unscented handcream or foot lotion.

Hands:
  Camomile, lavender, benzoin.

Feet:
  Sandalwood, lavender, rosewood.
  (For tired hot feet: a few drops of peppermint is wonderfully cooling.)

HAIRCARE

There's no better sign of good health than a shiny head of glossy hair and yet hair driers, bleaching, colouring, pollution, cheap shampoos, sun and sea all affect the condition. As with other areas of beauty, the essential oils can be added to your favourite brands as this will help boost their effectiveness or add to unscented shampoos available from essential oil suppliers or health shops.

Normal:
  Rosemary, lavender, lemon, cedarwood, sandalwood.

Dry:
  Sandalwood, camomile, lavender, rosemary.

Greasy:
  Lemon, rosemary, cypress, geranium.

Dandruff:
  Rosemary, lemon, eucalyptus, tea tree (although tea tree is effective, some people are put off by the overpowering smell of disinfectant in which case it is advisable to scent your products with preferred fragrances).

Balding:

Add a few drops of cedarwood and rosemary oil to shampoo and conditioner, plus give the scalp regular vigorous massage with a base oil containing the above mentioned two essential oils – 3% essential to 97% base oil will be sufficient.

To enhance hair colour, add 6 drops of essential oil to the final rinse.

Dark hair:

Rosemary, cedarwood.

Fair hair:

Lemon, camomile.

MONTHLY TREATMENT

Add the appropriate essential oil to a base oil. Part the hair and apply the oil from the roots of the hair to the ends. Wrap the head in a warm towel and leave for 15 minutes. Shampoo thoroughly to remove all excess oil and you'll find that the hair will be left in a glossy, silky condition.

Greasy:

50 ml almond oil and 10 drops made up from lemon, rosemary, bergamot.

Dry:

50 ml almond oil and 10 drops made up from sandalwood, lavender, camomile.

Normal:

50 ml almond oil and 10 drops made up from rosewood, rosemary, lavender.

9

AN AID FOR WOMEN

A romatherapy can be used as an aid to women's health in a variety of ways. It can bring relief when suffering from minor disorders such as cystitis and thrush and it can help promote well-being and health during important times such as pregnancy, childbirth and postnatal.

WOMEN'S HEALTH

MINOR DISORDERS

Anyone who has suffered the discomfort of cystitis is probably familiar with the frustrating cycle it is easy to fall into. Often antibiotics are prescribed and indeed do help clear it up and alleviate painful symptoms. However, many women find that as a result of taking the antibiotics, they develop thrush. The essential oils can be of tremendous help with both conditions and are often sought as a natural alternative to antibiotics, if used correctly and early on in the condition.

CYSTITIS

This is caused by a bacterial infection in the bladder or kidneys. The symptoms are a constant feeling of needing to urinate then a burning sensation when water is passed. It can be extremely painful if left untreated and travels up to the kidneys where symptoms become more serious. Acute lower back pain is felt, sweating and nausea.

SOLUTION:

1) As soon as you feel the symptoms, drink as much water as you can – 6 – 8 glasses. If you can stomach it, add a tablespoon of bicarbonate of soda as this will help dilute the acidity in the bladder and bring relief when passing water. Camomile tea is non-irritative and will also bring relief.

2) You can now buy remedies for cystitis over the counter at the chemist's which will help alkalize the urine but it will also help if you drink plenty of water with one of these remedies.

3) Avoid sugar, coffee, alcohol and spices.

4) Use a hot water bottle to bring comfort to the lower back.

5) You can use any of the following essential oils in several ways: lavender, camomile, juniper, bergamot or sandalwood.
   - In an aromatic bath to bring relief to the area that is burning.
   - Add the oils to a bowl of warm water, soak some cotton wool in the water and use to wipe the area. As it is such a sensitive area only use one per cent essential oil to the water otherwise it may sting.
   - In a hot compress which is applied to the lower back to bring relief and comfort.

If there is blood in the urine, acute backache and/or fever, waste no time in going to the doctor. Although he may prescribe antibiotics to kill the infection, you can still use the oils to bring relief and boost the recovery procedure.

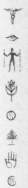

THRUSH

This is an infection caused by the fungus candida albicans. It usually affects the vaginal area though it can also affect the mouth, particularly in young babies. The symptoms are a discharge resembling cottage cheese accompanied by an unpleasant itching and sometimes by a stinging sensation when urinating.

The condition often occurs when rundown or following a course of antibiotics. As the antibiotics kill both good and bad bacteria in their task of eliminating infection, the result can be that in the intestines where everyone has candida, the intestinal interflora that usually keep the candida under control are no longer functioning so the candida proliferate and cause thrush. It can also be brought on by stress and women sufferers often find that they are more susceptible when they are fatigued.

Once candida has taken hold of a system it can be hard to get rid of and is very debilitating, not only because of the symptoms mentioned above but between the bouts of thrush the body may be left feeling bloated or tired. Here are some steps you can take to remedy it:

1) A visit to a nutritionist would be very helpful as they can prescribe vitamin and mineral supplements to help boost the system and a special diet for candida should be followed for between three to six months to rid the body and give the system a chance to regularize itself without the irritation of particular foods that candida loves and which help it to thrive.

2) Avoid starchy and sugary foods, fermented foods and anything with yeast in it.

3) Wear cotton underwear and loose fitting clothes.

4) Eat live yogurt which contains live bacteria which will help fight candida. Alternatively take acidiphollus tablets or lactobacillus capsules which replace the interflora that are supposed to be there naturally and so decrease the possibility of thrush happening. They are available from most health shops.

5) Don't use bubble baths as they can irritate and only use natural soaps.

6) You can use the following oils oils to alleviate some of the symptoms: lavender, myrrh, tea tree, bergamot or sandalwood.

- Daily baths/douches or sitz baths with 6–8 drops of the above oils.
- As described before for cystitis, as an essential oil wipe that has been soaked in warm water containing the oils.
- Soak a tampon in live yogurt to which has been added a drop of any of the above oils. Insert into the vagina and leave for half an hour.
- As stress is one of the causes of thrush, regular aromatherapy massage would help the system to relax and rejuvenate to the point that it can effectively fight infection again.

HERPES

Herpes is the same virus that produces cold sores. The symptoms are small blisterlike sores on the genitals that can sting and itch. The aromatherapy oils can be very effective in relieving the stinging and accelerating the recovery process.

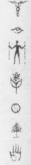

Oils to use are:

Tea tree, lavender, eucalyptus, lemon, sandalwood.

They can be used:

- In an aromatic bath.

- On cotton pads which have been soaked in warm water containing a few drops of the oils which are then used to wipe the area.

- Neat on a cotton bud which is then applied to the blister.

- As with thrush, herpes sufferers are often more susceptible when they are run down or under stress. If the stress is dealt with before it becomes a problem and the body is kept in peak condition, herpes is less likely to occur. Regular aromatherapy treatments could be an effective part of a lifestyle geared to prevent stress building to the point where it manifests physically.

PMT AND PERIOD PAINS

Women can suffer the effects of menstruation in several ways:

1) Premenstrual tension (PMT). Up to a week before the onset of menstruation, some women feel irrational, emotional, depressed, suffer mood swings, feel vulnerable or experience a lack of confidence. The following essential oils can help to redress the balance and can be used in a daily aromatic bath the week before the period or in a soothing massage a few days before the period when the symptoms appear:

    - For irritability: Sandalwood, rosewood, lavender, camomile
    - For depression: Ylang-ylang, clary sage, bergamot

- For mood swings: Geranium, sandalwood, rosewood
- For lack of confidence: Jasmine
- If feeling unattractive: Rose

2) Water retention. A few days before a period, many women experience feeling bloated as the body retains water. As some of the oils have diuretic properties, they can be used to alleviate this. They can be used in an aromatic bath or in a massage. (This would be most effective if it was received the day before the symptoms usually occur.)
   - For water retention: Juniper, clary sage, fennel, cypress.
   - Bloated feeling: Juniper, rosemary, cypress.

3) Painful menstruation. This can take the form of lower back pain, abdominal cramps and headaches.
   - Headaches: Peppermint, lavender.
   - Cramps: Camomile, lavender, clary sage, marjoram.
   - Lower back pain: Camomile, lavender.

The oils can be used in a bath or in a massage but particularly soothing for menstruation pain is a hot compress soaked in hot water containing the appropriate oils and placed on the abdomen or the lower back, then covered with a hot towel.

- For heavy periods: Cypress, rose or geranium can help normalize the flow and lavender or camomile will bring relief for the pain.
- For scanty, irregular periods: Clary sage, myrrh, sage, basil, juniper, fennel or rosemary will encourage the flow of menstrual blood. These oils should obviously be avoided if there is any chance of pregnancy.

THE MENOPAUSE

The change of life when women stop menstruating can happen any time from the forties to the late fifties and can be different for individual women. Just as some women don't experience any symptoms during menstruation so some women go through the menopause without any problems.

However, there are others for whom it can be difficult and their experiences can include hot flushes, moods swings, lack of confidence, dizziness, insomnia, fluid retention, irregular or scanty periods, sweating, depression and loss of sex drive.

As the symptoms are very similar to those experienced premenstrually and menstrually so are the oils that treat the discomfort experienced at the onset of the menopause.

The essential oils can be added to the bath or used in a base oil for body massage.

- For water retention and bloating: Juniper, fennel, rosemary.

- Feeling unattractive: Rose, jasmine.

- For a confidence boost: Jasmine.

- To regulate periods: Rose, geranium, cypress.

- For fatigue: Bergamot, rosemary.

- For insomnia: Marjoram, lavender.

- Lack of sex dive: Jasmine, clary sage, rose, sandalwood, ylang-ylang.

- Calming: Camomile, neroli.

- For balance: Geranium.

- Dizziness: Peppermint.

- Loss of concentration: Basil, peppermint.

- To soothe hot flushes: Geranium, camomile.

- For ageing, dry skin: Frankincense, neroli, rose, sandalwood, myrrh, patchouli

PREGNANCY

Throughout the pregnancy, essential oils can be of use, with different oils used at different stages. However, it is important to note that some of the oils should be avoided in pregnancy either because they are strong, too stimulating or are emmenagogue and will cause adverse reaction. (Oils that are emmenagogue are oils that encourage the flow of menstrual blood.) It is a good idea to register which these are and avoid them during the nine months.

Oils to avoid completely in pregnancy:

Aniseed, arnica, basil, camphor, clove, cypress, cinnamon, fennel, hyssop, juniper, marjoram, myrrh, sage, peppermint, rosemary, pennyroyal, myrrh, savory, sage, tarragon, thyme, nutmeg, origanum.

Oils to use with caution and not in the first stages:

Peppermint, clary sage, rose, jasmine, camomile.

DURING THE NINE MONTHS:

Pregnancy is a time when aromatherapy can be a tremendous aid both emotionally and physically. Most practitioners are trained to deal with pregnancy and booking regular sessions can bring help in several ways:

- To keep at bay the physical tension that can build in the neck and lower back.

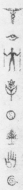

- To keep the circulation and lymph functioning efficiently.

- To take time to be pampered and rested.

- To help balance emotions that can feel unsteady in the light of such an overpowering experience of change.

- To relieve oedema (swollen legs or ankles).

A practitioner will help you choose oils that are going to be most beneficial for each individual pregnancy. As it effects every women differently, there is no one 'pregnancy formula' that is right for everyone.

Many of the oils that it is safe to use during pregnancy are the more sweetly scented ones and at a time when many smells, especially chemical or synthetic ones, can cause nausea, the essential oils, apart from their therapeutic value, offer much comfort by their fragrance.

Oils that are safe and can be use in an aromatic bath or gentle massage:

Bergamot – uplifting

Camomile (after first three months) – good for backache, muscle spasm, calming

Clary sage (at the birth) – can be used to induce labour and strengthen contractions

Geranium – balancing, soothes tenderness in breasts

Jasmine (after four months) – uplifting, effective for mood swings and postnatally for depression and to help restore balance

Lavender – good for headaches, backaches, calming, helps reduce high blood pressure

Lemon – refreshing tonic for the nervous system

Mandarin – good for stretchmarks

Neroli – good for stretchmarks, calming

Orange – good for constipation and stomach upsets

Patchouli – good for skincare if the skin has become dry, very relaxing

Rose (after four months) – good for dry skin, soothing, useful during the birth

Sandalwood – antiseptic, relaxing, good for urinary tract infections

Rosewood – good for skincare, reassuring and relaxing gentle scent

Tea tree – urinary tract infections, healing

Ylang-ylang – reduces high blood pressure and stress

For stretchmarks:

To prevent stretchmarks after the birth start your preventative measures early on in the pregnancy. A light base oil such as apricot kernel and oil of mandarin will do wonders to stop them ever appearing. 5 per cent essential oil to 95 per cent base oil will be sufficient. Apply every evening.

Labour:

Many women find using the aromatherapy oils to scent the labour or birth room very reassuring especially if away from home having a hospital birth. A few drops on a radiator will scent the atmosphere or alternatively if you want the scent to linger longer, wet a towel or flannel, sprinkle the drops of your

126 chosen oil and place on the radiator. If it is summer and no radiators will be on, it is an idea to invest in a burner (available at most health shops where essential oils are on sale or from one of the suppliers at the back of this book). Pack it ready in your bag for the hospital. Some oils you could use are:

Eucalyptus – cleans the air and aids breathing

Neroli – is very soothing and can act as a balm

Lavender – also smells clean and light

Oils to have ready for labour and the birth:
Clary sage – for its euphoric effect

Rose – as a uterine relaxant

Jasmine – to aid contractions

Neroli – calming

Nutmeg – primes the muscles for contractions

Lavender – relaxes

These oils can be diluted in a base oil and gently rubbed in to the lower back during labour or (as some women don't like to be touched during labour) in a warm compress applied to the abdomen or lower back.

For the breasts:
Fennel oil can help the flow of breast milk. It is advisable to apply it diluted in a base oil just prior to the birth and just afterwards to stimulate and promote a painless flow of milk.

Geranium oil in a base oil will help soothe swollen breasts. This can either be gently applied in a base oil or applied in a cool compress to reduce swelling.

For sore or cracked nipples a soothing remedy is a few drops of rose oil, a few drops of camomile in 2 teaspoons of almond oil. This will relieve dryness but it is important to cleanse the area afterwards with an unperfumed cleanser before breast-feeding.

POSTNATAL

As with the pregnancy and the birth, this can affect women in a variety of ways. Some can feel euphoric, others can dive into a severe depression that is hard to shake off, almost all experience fatigue.

It is a demanding time both emotionally and physically with more changes taking place as the body adjusts to no longer being pregnant (not to mention the demands of sleepless nights and adjusting to feeding and entertaining wide awake babies).

If it is possible to continue with aromatherapy treatments, they will be of great help as they give the new mother some time to recharge and rest at a time when it is sorely needed.

Oils that are beneficial postnatally for home use either in massage or in an aromatic bath are:

As a pick-me-up – rosemary/bergamot.

To heal – rose/camomile.

To aid sleep – lavender/marjoram.

To help milk flow – fennel.

For depression – jasmine, bergamot.

THE SENSUAL SIDE
TO AROMATHERAPY

As well as the many benefits attainable from the oils for medicinal and therapeutic purposes, they can also be used to enhance and improve the sensual and sexual side of life. We're living at a time when statistics tell us that whilst one in three modern marriages ends in divorce, the average couple makes love three times a week. Between these two statistics is enough pressure to 'get it right' to cause even the best partnership to break down. What if you don't make love that often, is it going to be divorce? Although it is true that some of the oils do have aphrodisiac properties, it isn't a question of adding a few drops here and all will be well (whatever that means for you). The aromatherapy approach is always to look at things holistically. There are many factors that can affect someone's love life and all these could be looked at and helped with the use of the essential oils.

STRESS

Stress is one of the prime causes of a diminished libido. Anxiety about work, financial worry, insecurity, all take their toll and end up like a huge dampener that can block any sexual feeling especially if even your time off is fraught with tension that is hard to shake off.

The best way to deal with a lack of desire in this instance is to go to the root of the problem and alleviate the stress and aromatherapy is one of the most effective treatments for doing this. Once a person is more relaxed physically and mentally, although perhaps the external problems won't have gone away, they will be better equipped to deal with them.

Once things are more in perspective, it will be easier to let the deeper feelings that have been blocked to come to the surface and with them the re-emergence of sexuality. Oils that are good for stress are lavender, neroli, sandalwood, bergamot (see also Chapter 6 on stress). Marjoram though good for stress is actually an anti-aphrodisiac so in this case, it would be advisable to use one of the above oils.

LACK OF CONFIDENCE

With magazines full of beautiful models both male and female, many people feel that they don't quite match up. They have a negative body image and feel shy or inhibited about taking their clothes off and enjoying free lovemaking. The oils best for this would be all of the oils that uplift and evoke a sense of well-being and inner beauty. These would be best used in the beginning of a relationship either in the bath or a non-sexual massage.

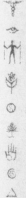

If someone isn't used to physical contact, a gentle non-sexual massage is a good way for a couple to get to know each other and get used to each other's touch. For men in particular, so much of the time, there is an unspoken pressure to be a good lover and perform well. To relax and enjoy the sensation of a gentle massage with no expectations sexually can remove a lot of this tension.

Oils:

Ylang-ylang – uplifting, mellowing.

Jasmine – gives a sense of joy and inner confidence.

Rose – a sense of lightness and femininity.

Sandalwood – relaxing.

Bergamot – uplifting and light.

FATIGUE

Fatigue is also high on the list of passion killers. In this case, oils that stimulate and awaken would be most beneficial. Try a combination of:

Black pepper, lemon and sandalwood or

Ginger, bergamot and sandalwood,

Jasmine, lemon, black pepper

Ylang-ylang, black pepper, ginger

HEALTH

A healthy libido is a sign of good health. If due to a fast and stressful lifestyle your health has deteriorated, it will also affect your sex drive. A change of diet, a tonic for being rundown with vitamin and mineral supplements, a weekend off, fresh air and gentle exercise will all contribute to bringing back sexual desire. The oils that could help would be the ones to strengthen, refresh and revive.

Oils:

Try one of the following combinations in the bath or in a massage:

Cinnamon, lemon, ginger

Rosemary, bergamot, sandalwood

Bergamot, black pepper, cedarwood

LACK OF EXERCISE

This can result in a general feeling of sluggishness and lack of sexual desire. A gentle exercise programme to start with could be combined with the use of stimulating oils to revive your system back into a feeling of well-being and healthy libido.

Oils:

Peppermint, bergamot, lemon, ginger, rosemary are all refreshing and reviving.

LACK OF COMMUNICATION

This is perhaps the greatest cause of break-ups. If communication breaks down between a couple because minor misunderstandings and resentments never get voiced, the deeper feelings of love and desire get buried beneath until it seems that they are hardly there. Women in particular find it hard to feel sexual with their partner if petty grievances haven't been resolved. As sexuality involves being open and vulnerable with a partner, it is easier to do so if everything is clear between you.

The essential oils and the use of massage can help with this as the first step. The physical contact of massage, even non-sexual, can sometimes allow deeper feelings to surface and can help move towards verbal communication. Once that is established again then sexual contact is more likely.

Oils:

> Clary sage – to uplift and disperse anger.
>
> Frankincense – helps the heart to open and aids communication.
>
> Neroli – can calm a tense situation.
>
> Sandalwood – can relax and dissolve feelings of bitterness.
>
> Rose – can heal rifts.
>
> Geranium – will help restore balance.
>
> Rosewood – to reassure.

BRIDGING THE GAP

Even if things are good between a couple, they are still often up against the everyday survival of ordinary living. Journeys home fraught with delay, children who won't go to sleep and have been demanding, all the various elements that don't exactly put a person in the frame of mind for sex.

The aphrodisiac oils can help bridge the various gaps we all have in our lives between our public faces of coping and surviving and the more private face where we feel free to be intimate and relaxed enough to let the barriers down.

Here, the oils with the aphrodisiac properties can be used to create a mood of sensuality in three ways:

1) As mood enhancers: The scent of the aphrodisiac oils can be used to create ambiance. All of us are affected by the five senses, sight, sound, feeling, taste and smell and all of these should be addressed as part of our sensual life. Sadly

though, the sense of smell often comes last if it is not neglected altogether. The oils can be used to arouse this powerful sense with their evocative fragrance.

You can burn the oils in burners available from most health shops or on the radiator as described in Chapter 3.

Try jasmine or sandalwood on their own.

Ylang-ylang and patchouli for an exotic scent.

Rose and rosewood for a delicate warm scent.

Cinnamon, orange and frankincense for a spicy fragrance.

Bergamot, orange and rosewood for a warm, cosy scent.

2) Use any of the following oils: Ylang-ylang, clary sage, rose, jasmine, sandalwood, patchouli, all of which have aphrodisiac properties in an aromatic bath to help shake off the day's responsibilities and change your mood into one of lazy relaxation.

3) In a base oil for a massage. You could use any of the aphrodisiac oils: ylang-ylang, clary sage, rose, jasmine, sandalwood, patchouli, either on their own or in combination with any of the following which are warming and stimulating: black pepper, cinnamon, coriander, cardamon, ginger.

For example:

Jasmine and ginger

Black pepper, jasmine and sandalwood

Rose and clary sage

Rose and cinnamon

Ylang-ylang and black pepper

Coriander, black pepper and ylang-ylang

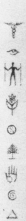

Do not use the essential oils directly on the sexual areas as they may sting.

PRINCIPLES OF AROMATHERAPY

RECIPES FOR SUCCESS: BLENDING THE OILS

B lending the oils for a pleasing scent as well as therapeutic benefit is something that will come as you experiment and become familiar with the various individual scents. Every aromatherapist has his or her own particular favourites which have come with using the oils over months or years. This can be confusing as if you read different books on aromatherapy or ask a few different practitioners what oils they would recommend for a particular condition it may seem like they're all contradicting each other by giving different answers. It isn't that one combination is better or right or wrong or that any one practitioner's choice is more informed. The oils are all versatile, so there is such a wide choice of oils for the same conditions that practitioners simply formulate their own favourites through experience. They may choose their particular combinations because of

A) The smell.

B) They feel certain oils are best therapeutically in a particular combination.

C) A particular combination suits a particular client's needs.

For the newcomer, it is a learning experience and an art in itself especially when it comes to combining the various scents from different families, for example a menthol with a flowery or a herbal with citrus or woody scent. It is here that you may run into trouble and sometimes end up with strange smelling concoctions. There are however some very simple tips to making successful and pleasing aromas and if you stick by them you'll find you have no problem.

THE THREE NOTES OF SCENT

According to the perfumers, there are three types of scent which they call notes and it is the combination of these that make a successful well-balanced perfume.

1) The top note. This is the scent that usually hits you first, it is the most volatile and also the quickest to disperse. Usually quite intense, it is either very sharp or very sweet. Examples: lemon, bergamot.

2) The middle note. This is exactly as described, a scent that is neither too light nor too heavy, resting in the middle, it will be detected under the immediate smell of the top note. Examples are lavender, black pepper.

3) The base. The heavy aroma that usually lingers longest. This scent is the slowest to disperse. It is the last to reach the nostrils and is the scent that can linger long after the other two have disappeared. Examples are cedarwood, patchouli. This base oil can also 'fix' the other notes, slowing down their volatility and giving the overall scent more staying power.

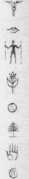

A combination of the three notes results in a scent that is neither too heavy nor too sharp but will be detected layer by layer as the different notes reach the nose. Having said all this, don't feel you have to stick to a rigid rule of three notes every time you blend. Sometimes your needs at a particular time will instinctively determine which oils you are drawn to. For example, when suffering from flu, the menthol scents may smell wonderful and yet so many of then are top notes. A combination of three top notes may not make a well-balanced scent to a perfumer but a sharp intense smell is just what you need at that time to cut through mucus and blocked sinuses. A week later when you have recovered, you may find the same oils too sharp and they do nothing for you scentwise.

Here is a chart detailing the note of each oil.

4

ESSENTIAL OIL	NOTE	SCENT TYPE
Angelica:	base	herb
Aniseed:	top	herb
Basil:	top	herb
Bay:	top	menthol
Benzoin:	base	woody
Bergamot:	top	citrus
Black Pepper:	middle	spice
Cajuput:	top	menthol
Camomile:middle	flower	herb
Camphor:	base	menthol
Caraway:	top	herb
Cardamom:	top	spice
Carrot seed:	middle	herb
Cedarwood:	base	woody
Celery:	middle	herb

Cinnamon:	base	spice
Citronella:	top	herb
Clary sage:	middle	herb
Clove:	base	spice
Coriander:	top	herb
Cumin:	top	spice
Cypress:	base/middle	woody
Eucalyptus:	top	menthol
Fennel:	middle	herby
Frankincense:	base	resin
Garlic:	middle	herb
Geranium:	middle	flower
Ginger:	middle	spice
Grapefruit:	top	citrus
Hyssop:	middle	herb
Jasmine:	middle	flower
Juniper:	middle	herb
Lavender:	middle	flower
Lemon:	top	citrus
Lemongrass:	top	herb
Lime:	top	citrus
Mandarin:	top	citrus
Marjoram:	middle	herb
Melissa:	middle	flowery herb
Myrrh:	base	resin
Neroli:	middle	flower
Niaouli:	top	menthol
Nutmeg:	top	spice
Orange:	top	citrus
Origanum:	middle	herb
Palmarosa:	top	herb
Parsley:	middle	herb
Patchouli:	base	woody
Peppermint:	top	menthol
Petitgrain:	middle	woody/flower

Pine:	middle	wood
Rose:	middle	flower
Rosemary:	middle	herb
Rosewood:	middle	woody
Sage:	top	herb
Sandalwood:	base	woody
Spearmint:	top	menthol
Tangerine:	top	citrus
Tarragon:	top	herb
Thyme:	top	herb
Tea tree:	top	disinfectant
Verbena:	top	herb
Vetivert:	base	woody
Ylang-ylang:	middle	flower

This is just meant as a guide to the different notes to help you select oils. You may find in different books on aromatherapy that there is some disagreement over a few oils as to whether they are top, base or middle notes. Certainly a few seem to hover on the borderline, in those cases, the best policy is simply to use your own nose and let that be the decider.

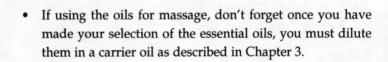

- If using the oils for massage, don't forget once you have made your selection of the essential oils, you must dilute them in a carrier oil as described in Chapter 3.

TIPS FOR MIXING

- Lemon and lavender are great for coming to the rescue of an aroma disaster. Both these two oils can even out a scent that is too overpowering and heavy or too light and sharp.

- Oils from the same family blend harmoniously. For example all the flowers – rose, geranium, jasmine; or all the herby ones – basil, rosemary, marjoram; or all the spices – cinnamon, ginger, black pepper; all the woods – rosewood, sandalwood.

- Spices and citrus blend well together, for example: ginger and lemon, cinnamon and orange, black pepper and lime.

- Woody scents and citrus also blend well, for example rosewood and bergamot, cedarwood and lime.

- Certain oils tend to take over any scent combination, these are peppermint, fennel, tea tree, clove, thyme, patchouli and camomile. Although the last two could easily be lightened with lemon.

- The menthol and the flowery scents don't tend to make a pleasing scent whatever the note combination, for example, peppermint and geranium, eucalyptus and orange, cajeput and ylang-ylang wouldn't smell good, at least to my taste.

- You don't always have to combine the oils for a pleasing scent. Many of them smell good on their own, for example jasmine, rose, neroli, orange, rosewood, ylang-ylang all stand up on their own.

- You don't have to always stick to three oils when mixing. It's just that mixing more than three, you have to know the individual scents well to avoid aroma disasters. On the other hand you don't have to use as many as three, in many cases two is quite sufficient for a pleasing scent.

As you become more confident, you will find your own combinations and preferences. With any art like cooking or painting,

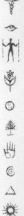

each individual makes their own choices. This is another aspect of aromatherapy, the chance to bring your own preferences into the process by choosing your own selection for different moods, needs or conditions.

In the meantime, here's a few examples to get you started. As you'll see, some conform to the three notes formula (an oil from the top, an oil from the middle and a base oil), some don't.

ANXIETY:

Neroli, petitgrain, sandalwood

APHRODISIAC:

Ylang-ylang, black pepper, sandalwood

Jasmine, lemon, sandalwood

Jasmine, clary sage, sandalwood

Rose, ylang-ylang, sandalwood

CELLULITE:

Juniper, black pepper, cypress

FOR CHRISTMAS,
TO WARM AND CREATE ATMOSPHERE:

Frankincense, lemon, myrrh

Cinnamon, orange, clove, sandalwood

Cinnamon, mandarin, nutmeg, sandalwood

CONVALESCENCE:

Cinnamon, lemon, ginger

Jasmine, lemon, sandalwood

Ylang-ylang, bergamot, rosewood

FATIGUE:

Bergamot, rosemary, ginger

Coriander, lemon, black pepper

Juniper, lime, rosemary

FLU:

Basil, eucalyptus, marjoram

Peppermint, rosemary, eucalyptus

HANGOVERS:

Juniper, lemon, rosemary

Bergamot, juniper, basil

Rosemary, fennel, lemon

INSOMNIA:

Marjoram, petitgrain, rosewood

Lavender, clary sage, sandalwood

Neroli, lavender, benzoin

JETLAG:

Bergamot, rosemary, sandalwood

MUSCLE ACHE:

Rosemary, juniper, ginger

Rosemary, petitgrain, lavender

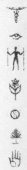

RELAXATION:

Rose, lavender, sandalwood

Geranium, lemon, rosewood

Neroli, petitgrain, sandalwood

STIMULANT:

Grapefruit, rosemary, ginger

Lime, black pepper, ginger

PURELY FOR SCENT:

Men's Preferences

Lime, lavender, cedarwood

Frankincense, lemon, vetivert

Neroli, lemon, sandalwood

Women's Preferences

Rose, lemon, sandalwood

Petitgrain, lemon, rosewood

Ylang-ylang, lemon, sandalwood

Cinnamon, lemon, sandalwood

POT POURRI:

Rose, frankincense, rosewood

Frankincense, orange, sandalwood

Lemongrass, rosemary, sandalwood

Jasmine, frankincense, sandalwood

Cedarwood, orange, cypress

Pine, rosemary, sandalwood

Neroli, rosewood, lemon

Cinnamon, clove, nutmeg, orange

SUMMER:
TO REFRESH AND COOL THE AIR

Bergamot and rosemary

Peppermint and basil

Lemongrass and rosemary

Lime, grapefruit, rosemary

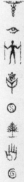

INDEX OF OILS AND USES

OIL	BOTANICAL NAME
Angelica:	Angelica archangelica
Used for:	coughs, colds, indigestion, fevers
Aniseed:	Pimpinella anisum
Used for:	coughs, catarrh, bronchitis, indigestion, circulation
Basil:	Ocimum Basilicum
Used for:	mental fatigue, bronchitis, migraine, gout, loss of concentration, colds, asthma, fainting
Bay:	Laurus Nobilis/Pimenta Racemosa
Used for:	colds, flu, rheumatism, sinusitis
Benzoin:	Styrax Benzoin
Used for:	coughs, colds, arthritis, sedative, digestive problems
Bergamot:	Citrus Bergamia
Used for:	acne, skin problems, herpes, tension, depression, stress, fevers, cystitis
Birch:	Betula Lenta
Used for:	ulcers, rheumatism, gout
Black Pepper:	Piper Nigrum
Used for:	colds, cellulite, flatulence, rheumatism, flu

Cajuput: Melaleuca cajeputi/leucadendron
Used for: flu, colds, colic, bronchitis, respiratory conditions, acne, psoriasis, cystitis
Camphor: Cinnamomum camphora
Used for: coughs, colds, fevers, rheumatism, arthritis
Caraway: Carum carvi
Used for: earache, vertigo, tonic, throat and chest problems, bruising
Cardamom: Elettaria Cardomomum
Used for: nausea, headaches, digestion, coughs
Carrot seed: Daucus carota
Used for: eczema, psoriasis, ulcers, diuretic
Cedarwood: Cedrus Atlantica
Used for: bronchitis, hair loss, catarrh, acne, diuretic, urinary problems
Celery: Apium Graveolens
Used for: diuretic, cellulite, rheumatism, arthritis, gout
Chamomile Roman: Ormensis Multicaulis
Used for: migraine, acne, inflammation, insomnia, menstrual problems, nerves, stress
Chamomile Blue: Matricaria Recutica
Used for: anxiety, menstrual problems, digestive/stomach disorders, inflammation
Cinnamon: Cinnamomum Zeylanicum
Used for: flu, rheumatism, coughs, colds, virus's, feeling the cold, appetite stimulant, circulation, convalescence
Citronella: Cymbopogon Nardus
Used for: stimulant, insect repellent
Clary sage: Salvia Sclarea
Used for: depression, nerves, menstrual problems, sedative, asthma, frigidity, impotence
Clove: Eugenia Caryophyllata
Used for: toothache, infection, nausea, flatulence, bronchitis, diarrhoea

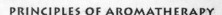

Coriander: Coriandrum Sativum

Used for: indigestion, fatigue, rheumatism, flu, constipation, flatulence

Cumin: Cuminum Cyminum

Used for: headaches, indigestion, liver problems

Cypress: Cupressus Sempervirens

Used for: circulation, rheumatism, colds, coughs, wounds, menopausal problems, haemorrhoids, asthma, wounds

Dill: Anethum graveolens

Used for: indigestion, constipation,

Elemi: Canarium Commune/luzonicum

Used for: colds, ulcers, wounds, congested lungs

Eucalyptus: Eucalyptus Globulus/Citriodora

Used for: coughs, bronchitis, sore throat, sinusitis, rheumatism, skin infections, viral infections, migraine, herpes, mosquito repellent, strained muscles

Fennel: Foeniculum Vulgare

Used for: digestive problems, constipation, diuretic, menopausal problems, kidney stones, flatulence, postnatal (it helps the flow of milk in case of any congestion)

Frankincense: Boswellia Thurfera/Carteri

Used for: chest complaints, coughs, bronchitis, wounds, colds,nerve tonic, skincare (it helps keep ageing skin younger)

Galbanum: Ferula galbaniflua

Used for: bronchitis, inflammations, encourages scar tissue to heal

Garlic: Allium sativum

Used for: asthma, coughs colds, wounds, insect bites, ulcers, decongestant

Geranium: Pelargonium Graveolens

Used for: tonic, balancing, depression, menstrual problems, eczema, neuralgia, circulatory problems, mastitis, chilblains, mosquito repellent

Ginger: Zingiber Officinale
Used for: colds, nausea, digestive problems, rheumatism, muscular aches and pains, sprains, appetite loss, flatulence, convalescence

Grapefruit: Citrus Paradisi
Used for: tonic, depression, liver and kidney problems

Hyssop: Hyssopus Officinalis
Used for: rheumatism, bruises, coughs, colds, viral infections, circulatory problems, asthma, hayfever

Jasmine: Jasminum Officinale/graniflorum
Used for: depression, menstrual problems, stress, skincare (dry skin) postnatal depression

Juniper: Juniperus Communis
Used for: liver problems, acne, urinary infections, diuretic, obesity, appetite stimulant, period pains, eczema, psoriasis, ulcers, wounds, detoxifying, hangovers

Lavender: Lavandula Vera/Augustifolium/Officinalis
Used for: burns, skin infections, cuts, wounds, eczema, dermatitis, flu, nausea, stress, headaches, asthma, rheumatism, arthritis, cystitis, high blood pressure, muscle spasm, sunburn, fainting

Lemon: Citrus Limonum
Used for: digestive problems, sore throat, as a nervous tonic, skin problems, insect repellent, arthritis, lowers blood pressure

Lemongrass: Cybopogon Citratus
Used for: chest problems, insect repellent, headaches, sore throat, insufficient milk after birth, blocked intestines

Lime: Citrus Aurantifolia
Used for: sore throats, tonic, fevers, rheumatism, headaches, alcoholism

Linden Blossom: Tilia Cordata/europaea
Used for: tonic, headaches, migraine, vertigo, neuralgia, catarrh, flu, mouth ulcers, respiratory conditions

148

Mandarin:	Citrus mandurensis/reticulata
Used for:	anxiety, tranquillizer, digestive problems, insomnia, stretchmarks, liver problems, skincare (oily skin)
Marjoram:	Thymus Masticana/Origanum Majorana
Used for:	sprains, bruises, colds, rheumatism, menstrual problems, bronchitis, insomnia, constipation, asthma, flatulence
Melissa:	Melissa Officinalis
Used for:	anxiety, bacterial or fungal infections, eczema, sedative, allergies, menstrual problems, asthma
Myrrh:	Commiphora Myrrha
Used for:	wounds, mouth ulcers, bacterial infections, fungal infections, candida, bronchitis, laryngitis, skincare, menstrual problems, catarrh,
Myrtle:	Myrtus communis
Used for:	asthma, digestion, respiratory problems
Neroli:	Citrus Aurantium
Used for:	depression, anxiety, cardiac, diarrhoea, menopausal problems, skincare, lowers high blood pressure, acne, eczema, insomnia
Niaouli:	Melaleuca Virdiflora
Used for:	respiratory problems, sore throats, burns, acne, cuts and wounds, cystitis, strengthens the immune system, diarrhoea
Nutmeg:	Myristica Fragrans
Used for:	nausea, rheumatism, arthritis, insomnia, respiratory problems, acne
Orange:	Citrus cinensis
Used for:	constipation, sedative, stomach problems, tranquillizing
Oregano:	Origanum vulgare
Used for:	bronchitis, viral infections, rheumatism, digestive problems, loss of appetite
Palmarosa:	Cymbopogon Martini
Used for:	tonic, skin infections

Parsley: Petroselinum sativum

Used for: menstrual problems, menopausal problems, diuretic, kidney problems

Patchouli: Pogostemon Patchouli

Used for: skin infections and problems, acne, eczema, fungal infections, diuretic, anxiety

Peppermint: Mentha Piperascens

Used for: nausea, travel sickness, headaches, flu, migraine, fevers, inflammation, arthritis, sinusitis, painful periods, mosquito repellent

Petitgrain: Citrus Aurantium

Used for: anxiety, depression, stress, insomnia, convalescence

Pimento: Pimento officinalis

Used for: indigestion, colds, rheumatism, muscular strains, depression, circulation, cramps

Pine: Pinus Sylvestris

Used for: chest infections, colds, coughs, catarrh, bladder and kidney infections, circulation, muscular aches and pains, sore throats

Rose: Rosa Damascena/centifolia

Used for: stress, menopausal problems, constipation, skincare, grief, nausea

Rosemary: Rosmarinus Officinalis

Used for: headaches, muscular strains, fatigue, dandruff, alopecia, stimulant, liver decongestant

Rosewood: Aniba Rosaedora

Used for: skin allergies, depression, stress, headaches

Sage: Salvia officinalis

Used for: bronchitis, catarrh, rheumatism, arthritis, fibrositis, insect bites or stings, eczema, candida

Sandalwood: Santalum Album

Used for: acne, catarrh, sore throat, cystitis, menstrual problems, skin infections, fungal and bacterial problems, eczema, skincare

Spearmint: Mentha Spicata
Used for: indigestion, intestinal cramps, fever, nausea, haemorrhoids, bad breath

Tangerine: Citrus Reticulata
Used for: rheumatism, cellulite, stretchmarks, tonic, stomach problems

Tarragon: Artemisia dracunculus
Used for: diuretic, wounds, rheumatism, arthritis, laxative, calms menstrual pain

Thyme: Thymus Vulgaris
Used for: bacterial and urinary infections, rheumatism, viral infection, wounds, hair loss, gum and teeth care, fatigue, difficult periods

Tea tree: Melaleuca Alternifolia
Used for: fungal infections, viral and bacterial infections, colds, flu, cold sores, acne, candida, burns, athlete's foot, insect repellent

Verbena: Lippia citriodora
Used for: tonic, digestive complaints, asthmatic coughs

Vetivert: Vetivera Zizanoides/Andropogan muricatus
Used for: stress, insomnia, rheumatism, respiratory complaints

Violet: Viola odorata
Used for: kidney problems, skin infections, rheumatism, liver decongestant

Yarrow: Achillea millefolium
Used for: cramps, inflammation, constipation, circulation, menstrual problems

Ylang-ylang: Cananga Odorata
Used for: anxiety, lowers high blood pressure, depression, aphrodisiac, regulates and calms the heart, skincare

INDEX OF COMMON
AILMENTS AND THE OILS
AND METHODS OF USE

Abcesses/boils: camomile, lavender, bergamot, juniper, tea tree, clary sage.
Method of application: compress
Acne: sandalwood, lemon, bergamot, juniper, lavender, geranium, myrrh, petitgrain, tea tree
Method of application: compress or in skin products
Ageing skin: frankincense, myrrh, rose, patchouli, lavender, lemon, carrot, neroli
Method of application: beauty mask, added to oil based skin products
Allergies: camomile, melissa, lavender
Method of application: inhalation/massage
Alcoholism: fennel, juniper (detoxifying)
Method of application: aromatic bath
Alopecia: cedarwood, clary sage, rosemary, lavender, thyme, pimento
Method of application: massage, water rinse, added to hair products
Amenorrhoea: clary sage, lavender, camomile, cypress, parsley
Method of application: compress/massage/aromatic bath
Anxiety: benzoin, bergamot, camomile, clary sage, cedarwood, cypress, frankincense, geranium, jasmine, juniper, neroli, lavender, vetivert, rosewood, rose, sandalwood, patchouli, mandarin, melissa, marjoram, ylang-ylang
Method of application: massage/aromatic bath

Appetite loss: bergamot, camomile, ginger, cinnamon, fennel, mint, cardoman
Method of application: massage
Arthritis: juniper, fennel, rosemary, lemon, eucalyptus, ginger, camomile, lavender, cypress, cajuput, benzoin, black pepper
Method of application: massage, aromatic bath
Asthma: bergamot, camomile, lavender, cypress, eucalyptus, marjoram, melissa, basil, myrtle, frankincense, thyme
Method of application: inhalation/massage
Athlete's foot: tea tree, lavender, myrrh, myrtle
Method of application: massage

Backache: lavender, rosemary, marjoram, ginger
Method of application: massage/aromatic bath
Baldness: cedarwood, rosemary
Method of application: in hair products/massage
Bedsores: camomile, lavender, geranium, patchouli
Method of application: compress/massage
Bleeding: lemon, cypress, geranium, rose, eucalyptus
Method of application: compress
Boils: camomile, lavender, bergamot, juniper, clary sage
Method of application: compress
Bronchitis: basil, benzoin, frankincense, lavender, peppermint, rosemary, eucalyptus, camphor, sandalwood, pine, bay, cajuput, origanum
Method of application: inhalation/massage
Bruises: lavender, camphor, cypress, hyssop
Method of application: compress
Burns: lavender, camomile, geranium, patchouli, benzoin
Method of application: compress

Candida: (see thrush)
Catarrh: cajuput, eucalyptus, lavender, niaouli, pine, rosemary, thyme
Method of application: inhalation

Cellulite: juniper, black pepper, clary sage, cypress, fennel, geranium, lemon, rosemary, tangerine
Method of application: massage/aromatic bath/compress

Chapped skin: benzoin, camomile, lavender
Method of application: compress/massage

Chest infections: eucalyptus, pine, benzoin, cajuput
Method of application: inhalation/massage

Chicken pox: camomile, lavender, eucalyptus, bergamot, tea tree
Method of application: aromatic bath/compress

Chilblains: cypress, black pepper, marjoram, rosemary, juniper, tea tree
Method of application: massage/aromatic bath

Circulatory problems: black pepper, cypress, lavender, juniper, sage, ylang ylang, marjoram, rosemary, cedarwood, geranium
Method of application: massage/aromatic bath

Colds: basil, camphor, cajuput, bay, niaouli, eucalyptus, lavender, tea tree, rosemary, garlic, hyssop, peppermint
Method of application: inhalation/massage

Cold sores: tea tree, lavender
Method of application: compress

Conjunctivitis: camomile, rose, lavender
Method of application: compress

Constipation: black pepper, bergamot, fennel, rose, juniper, lemongrass, rosemary, coriander, orange, marjoram
Method of application: massage

Convalescence: cinnamon, bergamot, ginger, petitgrain, rosemary
Method of application: massage/aromatic bath

Colitis: camomile
Method of application: compress/gentle massage

Coughs: benzoin, frankincense, eucalyptus, myrrh, rosemary, cypress, peppermint, pine, thyme
Method of application: inhalation/massage

Cramp: camomile, lavender, geranium, rosemary, sandalwood
Method of application: massage, compress

Cystitis: bergamot, cajuput, rose, lavender, juniper, sandalwood, cedarwood, pine, camomile
Method of application: massage/aromatic bath/douche

Dandruff: lemon, tea tree, rosemary, cedarwood
Method of application: in hair products/rinse water
Depression: basil, bergamot, clary sage, jasmine, geranium, rosewood, neroli, rose, sandalwood, ylang-ylang, melissa
Method of application: massage/aromatic bath/inhalation
Dermatitis: benzoin, camomile, frankincense, geranium, juniper, lavender, lemon, neroli, nutmeg
Method of application:massage/aromatic bath
Diarrhoea: black pepper, camomile, camphor, cypress, marjoram, niaouli, peppermint, rosemary, sandalwood, fennel, benzoin
Method of application: massage/aromatic bath/compress
Diuretic: fennel, juniper, clary sage, cypress, eucalyptus
Method of application: massage/aromatic bath
Dry skin: sandalwood, rose, lavender, geranium,
Method of application: massage/in skin products
Dysentery: black pepper, camomile, cypress
Method of application:compress/massage

Earache: camomile, lavender
Method of application:compress
Eczema: bergamot, camomile, lavender, geranium, hyssop, juniper, melissa, carrot
Method of application: massage/compress/aromatic bath
Exhaustion: rosemary, bergamot
Method of application: massage/aromatic bath

Fainting: basil, rosemary, peppermint, lavender, neroli
Method of application: inhalation
Fatigue: rosemary, geranium, basil, bergamot, peppermint, pine
Method of application: massage/aromatic bath/inhalation

Fever: basil, camomile, cypress, bergamot, juniper, lavender, melissa, eucalyptus, lavender, rosemary
Method of application: aromatic bath
Flatulence: black pepper, camomile, cardamom, ginger, fennel, juniper, lemongrass, peppermint, rosemary, coriander
Method of application: massage/compress
Frigidity: clary sage, rose, ginger, ylang ylang, cinnamon, sandalwood
Method of application: massage/aromatic bath

Gallstones: rosemary, lavender
Method of application: massage
Gingivitis: (inflamed gums) fennel, myrrh, thyme
Method of application: mouthwash
Gonorrhoea: bergamot, cedarwood
Method of application: massage/aromatic bath
Gout: basil, benzoin, camphor, lavender, juniper, rosemary,
Method of application: massage/compress
Grief: bergamot, rose, melissa, lavender, rosewood
Method of application: massage/aromatic bath
Gum disease: clove, clary sage
Method of application: mouthwash, apply with clean finger or cotton bud

Haemorrhoids: cypress, frankincense, juniper, myrrh, lavender, rosemary, myrtle
Method of application: massage/aromatic bath
Halitosis: spearmint, bergamot, nutmeg, cardamom, peppermint, myrrh
Method of application: mouthwash
Hangover: juniper, rosemary,
Method of application: massage/aromatic bath
Hayfever: eucalyptus, rose, lavender, melissa, camomile, pine, tea tree
Method of application: inhalation
Headaches: peppermint, lavender, marjoram, rose, lavender, rosemary, eucalyptus, camomile
Method of application: compress/massage

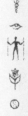

PRINCIPLES OF AROMATHERAPY

Heart: ylang-ylang, neroli, lavender, melissa
Method of application: massage/aromatic bath
Heartburn: cardamom, black pepper
Method of application: massage
Herpes: bergamot, patchouli, tea tree, lavender,
Method of application: compress
Hypertension: (high blood pressure) lavender, ylang-ylang, marjoram, camomile, neroli, bergamot, rose
Method of application: massage/aromatic bath
Hypotension: (low blood pressure) rosemary, camphor, peppermint, black pepper
Method of application: massage/aromatic bath
Hysteria: basil, clary sage, camomile, lavender, neroli, marjoram, melissa, ylang-ylang
Method of application: massage/aromatic bath/inhalation

Impetigo: benzoin, camomile, patchouli, lavender, tea tree
Method of application: aromatic bath/massage
Impotence: clary sage, jasmine, ginger, rose, sandalwood, ylang-ylang
Method of application: massage/aromatic bath
Indigestion: camomile, fennel, lavender, peppermint, basil, marjoram, coriander
Method of application: compress/massage
Inflammation: camomile, lavender
Method of application: compress
Influenza: black pepper, hyssop, niaouli, eucalyptus, rosemary, peppermint, garlic, tea tree, cypress
Method of application: aromatic bath/inhalation
Insect bites: lavender, eucalyptus, geranium
Method of application: compress
Insomnia: marjoram, lavender, camomile, neroli, sandalwood, petitgrain
Method of application: massage/aromatic bath
Irritability: lavender, camomile, neroli
Method of application: massage/aromatic bath

Itchiness: camomile, lavender, melissa, bergamot
Method of application: massage/compress

Jaundice: rosemary, camomile, thyme, peppermint
Method of application: massage/aromatic bath

Kidneys: juniper, sandalwood, fennel, camomile, cedarwood
Method of application: massage/aromatic bath/compress

Laryngitis: benzoin, sandalwood, lavender, frankincense, thyme, myrrh
Method of application: inhalation
Lice: lavender, lemon, geranium, eucalyptus
Method of application: aromatic bath/massage/scalp massage
Liver problems: juniper, lemon, cypress, rose, camomile, peppermint,
cumin, rosemary
Method of application: massage/aromatic bath/compress
Lumbago: juniper, rosemary, pine
Method of application: compress/massage

Mastitis: geranium, lavender, rose
Method of application: compress/massage
Measles: camomile, bergamot, eucalyptus, tea tree
Method of application: inhalation/aromatic bath
Memory (poor): basil, rosemary, peppermint
Method of application: inhalation
Menopause: camomile, lavender, rose, geranium, jasmine, bergamot,
clary sage, sandalwood, ylang-ylang
Method of application: massage/aromatic bath
Menstruation: rose, melissa, juniper, myrrh, clary sage, rosemary,
marjoram, camomile, cypress, pine
Method of application: compress/massage/aromatic bath
Mental fatigue: basil, rosemary, peppermint
Method of application: massage/aromatic bath/inhalation
Migraine: marjoram, peppermint, rosemary, camomile, lavender, basil
Method of application: massage/aromatic bath/inhalation

Mouth ulcers: myrrh, orange, tea tree
Method of application:mouthwash
Muscle strain: lavender, ginger, rosemary, juniper
Method of application: massage/aromatic bath

Nausea: basil, peppermint, lavender, fennel, rose, camomile, nutmeg, spearmint
Method of application: massage/aromatic bath/inhalation/compress
Nervous tension: benzoin, camomile, clary sage, lavender, neroli, patchouli, rose, sandalwood, ylang-ylang
Method of application: massage/aromatic bath
Nettle rash: camomile, melissa
Method of application: aromatic bath
Neuralgia: camomile, eucalyptus, geranium, lavender, marjoram, rosemary, clary sage, tea tree
Method of application: massage
Nose bleed: lemon, cypress, frankincense
Method of application: compress (cold)

Obesity: fennel, juniper, rosemary, lemon, bergamot, geranium
Method of application: massage/aromatic bath
Oedema: juniper, patchouli, fennel, geranium, lemon, rosemary, cypress, cedarwood
Method of application: massage/aromatic bath
Oily skin: bergamot, lemon, mandarin, sandalwood, geranium
Method of application: in skin preparations

Palpitations: camomile, lavender, orange, ylang-ylang, melissa, neroli, rosemary
Method of application: massage/inhalation
Pneumonia: cajuput, niaouli, pine, tea tree, eucalyptus, thyme
Method of application: inhalation/aromatic bath
Premenstrual tension: camomile, geranium, ylang-ylang, bergamot, rose, parsley
Method of application: massage/aromatic bath

Psoriasis: bergamot, benzoin, lavender, juniper, camomile, carrot
Method of application: compress/aromatic bath
Pyelitis: juniper, camomile, cedarwood, thyme
Method of application: massage

Relaxation: lavender, neroli, ylang-ylang, rosewood, marjoram, rose,
sandalwood, camomile, bergamot
Method of application: massage/aromatic bath
Rheumatism: rosemary, juniper, cypress, lavender, camomile, bay,
marjoram, coriander, cajuput, eucalyptus, lemon, sage, thyme, niaouli
Method of application: massage/aromatic bath
Ringworm: geranium, myrrh, lavender, rosemary, peppermint
Method of application: hair and skin preparations

Scabies: lavender, camomile, lemon, bergamot, rosemary, peppermint
Method of application: aromatic bath
Scalds: lavender, camomile, eucalyptus
Method of application: compress
Sciatica: camomile, lavender
Method of application: massage/aromatic bath/compress
Sensitive skin: camomile, neroli, rose, sandalwood
Method of application: massage/aromatic bath
Shingles: eucalyptus, geranium, bergamot, tea tree, peppermint, myrtle
Method of application: aromatic bath
Shock: camphor, neroli, peppermint
Method of application: inhalationpar Sinusitis: eucalyptus, lavender,
peppermint, niaouli, rosemary, bay, lavender, pine
Method of application: inhalation
Sinusitis: eucalyptus, lavender, peppermint, niaouli, rosemary, bay,
lavender, pine
Method of application: inhalation
Snakebite: lavender, tea tree, basil
Method of application: compress
Sore throat: lavender, sandalwood, benzoin, eucalyptus, niaouli, pine,
Method of application: inhalation/gargling

Sprains: eucalyptus, lavender, rosemary, camomile, marjoram
Method of application: compress (cold)
Stomach: fennel, peppermint, lavender, mandarin, orange, camomile
Method of application: compress/massage
Stress: bergamot, camomile, clary sage, marjoram, neroli, lavender, sandalwood, ylang-ylang, rose
Method of application: massage/aromatic bath
Stretchmarks: mandarin, tangerine
Method of application: massage
Sunburn: lavender, camomile
Method of application: compress/aromatic bath

Teething: camomile, lavender
Method of application: mouthwash/gentle massage
Thread veins: cypress
Method of application: massage
Throat: sandalwood, benzoin, tea tree
Method of application: mouthwash/gargle/inhalation
Thrush: myrrh, sandalwood, lavender, tea tree,
Method of application: douche/aromatic bath
Tonsillitis: lavender, benzoin
Method of application: inhalation/mouthwash (gargle)
Toothache: clove, camomile
Method of application: cotton bud compress
Travel sickness: peppermint
Method of application: inhalation

Ulcers: garlic
Method of application: compress
Urethritis: bergamot, lavender
Method of application: massage/aromatic bath

Varicose veins: cypress, geranium, lavender
Method of application: compress/massage
Vertigo: basil, rosemary, peppermint, black pepper
Method of application: inhalation
Viral Infections: bergamot, eucalyptus, tea tree,
Method of application: inhalation/aromatic bath
Vomiting: fennel, lavender, lemon, peppermint, rose, camomile
Method of application: compress

Warts: (verruca) tea tree, thuja, lemon
Method of application: compress
Water retention: geranium, juniper, parsley, fennel, pine, sage, violet leaves
Method of application: massage/aromatic bath
Whooping cough: basil, cypress, rosemary, niaouli, lavender, tea tree
Method of application: inhalation/massage
Worms: bergamot, camomile, eucalyptus, lavender
Method of application: massage/compress
Wounds: benzoin, lavender, eucalyptus, tea tree
Method of application: compress
Wrinkles: frankincense, lemon, sandalwood
Method of application: in skin preparations

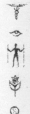

AN INDEX OF THE PROPERTIES OF THE OILS

PROPERTY	MEANING	OIL
Anaesthetic:	(insensitivity to pain)	cinnamon, clove, peppermint
Analgesic:	(pain relieving)	basil, bergamot, birch, black pepper, cajuput, camphor, camomile, clove, coriander, eucalyptus, galbanum, geranium, ginger, lavender, marjoram, niaouli, nutmeg, oregano, peppermint, pimento, rosemary
Anaphrodisiac:	(reduces sexual desire)	marjoram
Antacid:	(acid preventing)	lemon
Antiallergenic:	(reduces allergy symptoms)	camomile, melissa
Antibiotic:	(combats infection)	bergamot, camomile, cinnamon, clove, eucalyptus, garlic, hyssop, juniper, lavender, lemon, lime, myrtle, niaouli, nutmeg, origanum, patchouli, pine, tea tree, thyme

Anticoagulant:	(prevents or retards blood from clotting)	geranium
Anticonvulsive:	(prevents or retards convulsions)	camomile, clary sage, lavender
Antidepressant:	(uplifts, counteracts depression)	basil, bergamot, citronella, clary sage, geranium, grapefruit, jasmine, lavender, lemongrass, melissa, neroli, orange, patchouli, petitgrain, pimento, rose, rosemary, rosewood, ylang-ylang
Antidontalgic:	(helps relieve toothache)	cajuput, cinnamon, clove, nutmeg, peppermint
Antifungal:	(combats fungal diseases)	eucalyptus, juniper, lavender, lemon, myrtle, patchouli, pimento, sage, sandalwood, tea tree, thyme
Antineuralgic:	(reduces nerve pain)	bay, cajuput, clove, lemon
Antiphlogostic:	(reduces inflammation)	camomile, clary sage, eucalyptus, fennel, lavender, myrrh, patchouli, peppermint, pine, rose, sandalwood, yarrow
Antirheumatic:	(aids relief of rheumatism)	cajuput, camomile, cypress, eucalyptus, garlic, hyssop, juniper, lemon, lavender, niaouli, origanum, pine, rosemary, sage, tarragon, thyme
Antiseptic:	(cleans and fights infection)	all the oils are antiseptic
Antispasmodic:	(relieves cramp)	angelica, aniseed, basil, bergamot, bay, black pepper, cajuput, camomile, caraway, cardamom, camphor,

clary sage, clove, coriander,
dill, eucalyptus, fennel,
ginger, jasmine, juniper,
hyssop, lavender, mandarin,
marjoram, neroli, nutmeg,
orange, origanum, parsley,
peppermint, petitgrain, rose,
rosemary, sage, sandalwood,
spearmint, tangerine, thyme,
verbena, yarrow

Antivenomous: (neutralizes poison) basil, thyme

Antiviral: (controls virus) cinnamon, clove, elemi,
eucalyptus, garlic, lavender,
lime, oregano, palmarosa,
sandalwood, tea tree, thyme

Aperitif: (stimulates appetite) bay, caraway, cardamom,
cinnamon, clove, fennel,
ginger, nutmeg, origanum,
sage, thyme, tarragon

Aphrodisiac: (stimulates sexual desire) angelica, aniseed, basil,
black pepper, cardamom,
cinnamon, clary sage, clove,
cumin, ginger, jasmine,
juniper, nutmeg, neroli,
parsley, patchouli, pimento,
rose, rosewood, sandalwood,
thyme, verbena, vetivert,
violet, ylang-ylang

Astringent: (causes body tissue to
contract/tighten) bay, benzoin, birch, caraway,
cedarwood, cypress,
frankincense, geranium,
hyssop, juniper, lemon, lime,
myrrh, myrtle, patchouli,
peppermint, rose, rosemary,
sage, sandalwood, yarrow

Bacteriacide:	(combats bacteria)	basil, cumin, elemi, garlic, eucalyptus, lavender, lemon, lemongrass, lime, myrrh, myrtle, neroli, niaouli, palmarosa, rose, rosewood, tea tree
Balsamic:	(soothing)	cajuput, clary sage, elemi, eucalyptus, myrrh, niaouli, pine, tea tree
Bechic:	(relieves coughs)	ginger, hyssop, linden blossom, origanum, sandalwood, thyme
Cardiac:	(stimulates the heart)	aniseed, black pepper, caraway, camphor, cinnamon, hyssop, nutmeg, thyme
Carminative:	(cures flatulence)	angelica, aniseed, basil, bergamot, black pepper, caraway, cardamom, carrot seed, camomile, cinnamon, clove, coriander, cumin, dill, fennel, galbanum, ginger, hyssop, juniper, lemon, lemongrass, marjoram, melissa, myrtle, nutmeg, orange, origanum, parsley, peppermint, pimento, rosemary, spearmint, tarragon, thyme
Cephalic:	(clears the mind)	basil, cardamom, hyssop, marjoram, peppermint, rosemary, rosewood
Cordial:	(heart tonic)	benzoin, bergamot, lavender, marjoram, melissa, neroli, peppermint, rosemary, tea tree

Cytophylactic:	(encourages growth of new cells)	carrot, frankincense, geranium, lavender, mandarin, palmarosa, neroli, rose, tangerine
Decongestant:	(reduces and relieves mucus)	cajuput, eucalyptus, garlic, lavender, linden blossom, niaouli, peppermint, pine
Depurative:	(purifies the blood)	birch, caraway, carrot, coriander, cumin, eucalyptus, juniper, lemon, parsley, rose, sage
Detoxicant:	(neutralizes toxins)	black pepper, fennel, rose, sage
Digestive:	(aids digestion)	aniseed, basil, bergamot, black pepper, caraway, cardamom, camomile, clary sage, cumin, dill, lemongrass, mandarin, marjoram, melissa, neroli, orange, parsley, rosemary, tarragon, verbena
Disinfectant:	(destroys germs)	birch, caraway, clove, dill, juniper, lime, myrrh, pine
Diuretic:	(causes increased elimination of urine)	angelica, bay, benzoin, birch, black pepper, carrot, cedarwood, celery, camomile, cypress, eucalyptus, fennel, frankincense, galbanum, garlic, geranium, hyssop, juniper, lavender, lemon, lemongrass, linden blossom, parsley, patchouli, pine, rose, rosemary, sage, sandalwood, violet, yarrow
Emetic:	(causes vomiting)	rose, violet

Emmenagogue:	(encourages menstrual flow)	angelica, basil, bay, caraway, carrot, camomile, cinnamon, clary sage, cumin, fennel, galbanum, hyssop, jasmine, lavender, marjoram, myrrh, nutmeg, origanum, parsley, peppermint, rose, rosemary, sage, thyme
Emollient:	(soothing/softening)	cedarwood, camomile, geranium, jasmine, lavender, linden blossom, mandarin, rose, sandalwood, tangerine, verbena
Expectorant:	(clears lungs and chest)	angelica, basil, benzoin, bergamot, cajuput, camphor, cedarwood, elemi, eucalyptus, fennel, galbanum, garlic, ginger, hyssop, marjoram, myrrh, myrtle, origanum, parsley, peppermint, pine, sandalwood, tea tree, thyme, violet, yarrow
Febrifuge:	(dispels fever/cooling)	basil, bay, bergamot, cajuput, camphor, camomile, cypress, eucalyptus, garlic, ginger, hyssop, lemon, melissa, niaouli, orange, palmarosa, patchouli, peppermint, verbena
Fungicide:	(destroys fungal infections)	cedarwood, elemi, garlic, lavender, lemongrass, myrrh, patchouli, tea tree
Galactogenic:	(induces the flow of breast milk)	aniseed, basil, caraway, dill, fennel, jasmine, lemongrass

Haemostatic:	(stops or retards bleeding)	cinnamon, cypress, geranium, lemon, lime, rose
Hepatic:	(stimulates and encourages liver and gall bladder)	angelica, bay, carrot, camomile, cypress, grapefruit, lemon, origanum, peppermint, rose, sage, rosemary, verbena, violet
Hypertensive:	(increases blood pressure)	camphor, hyssop, rosemary, sage, thyme
Hypoglycemiant:	(lowers blood sugars)	eucalyptus, garlic, geranium
Hypotensive:	(lowers blood pressure)	celery, clary sage, garlic, lavender, lemon, linden blossom, marjoram, melissa, ylang-ylang
Insecticide:	(kills/repels insects)	aniseed, bay, bergamot, birch, cajuput, caraway, cedarwood, cinnamon, citronella, clove, cypress, eucalyptus, fennel, garlic, geranium, juniper, lemon, lemongrass, lime, myrtle, niaouli, origanum, patchouli, pine, tea tree, thyme
Laxative:	(causes bowels to evacuate)	aniseed, black pepper, camphor, fennel, ginger, lemon, marjoram, nutmeg, origanum, parsley, rose, tarragon, violet
Nervine:	(aids nervous disorders)	basil, camomile, clary sage, hyssop, juniper, lavender, linden blossom, marjoram, melissa, peppermint, rosemary, sandalwood, vetivert

Parasiticide:	(destroys parasites)	aniseed, caraway, cinnamon, citronella, clove, cumin, eucalyptus, garlic, lemon, lemongrass, myrtle, origanum, peppermint, rosemary, thyme
Parturient:	(aids childbirth)	aniseed, bay, clary sage, clove, dill, jasmine, juniper, lavender, nutmeg, parsley, rose, spearmint
Pectoral:	(helps diseases of chest and lungs)	cajuput, hyssop, violet
Prophylactic:	(helps prevent disease)	garlic, hyssop, lemongrass
Resolvent:	(reduces swellings)	fennel, galbanum, garlic, grapefruit, rosemary
Restorative:	(helps restore good health)	basil, cypress, lavender, lime, marjoram, pine, spearmint
Rubefacient:	(warming by increasing blood flow)	black pepper, camphor, eucalyptus, ginger, juniper, origanum, pimento, pine,
Sedative:	(calming, reduces excitement)	benzoin, bergamot, cedarwood, celery, camomile, clary sage, cypress, frankincense, geranium, jasmine, lavender, linden blossom, mandarin, marjoram, melissa, myrrh, neroli, petitgrain, rose, sage, sandalwood, verbena, vetivert, ylang-ylang
Splenetic:	(spleen tonic)	angelica, camomile, clove, fennel, origanum, lavender, rose

Stimulant:	(increases energy)	angelica, aniseed, basil, bay, black pepper, cajuput, camphor, caraway, cardamom, cinnamon, citronella, clove, coriander, cumin, eucalyptus, fennel, ginger, hyssop, lemongrass, niaouli, nutmeg, origanum, peppermint, pine, rosemary, spearmint, tarragon, thyme
Stomachic:	(good for the stomach)	angelica, aniseed, basil, bay, bergamot, black pepper, cardamom, camomile, cinnamon, clary sage, clove, coriander, dill, fennel, ginger, hyssop, juniper, lemon, melissa, myrrh, nutmeg, orange, origanum, peppermint, pimento, rose, rosemary, tangerine, tarragon, verbena
Styptic:	(stops external bleeding)	cypress, lemon
Sudorific:	(promotes perspiration)	angelica, basil, cajuput, camphor, camomile, dill, fennel, garlic, ginger, melissa hyssop, juniper, lavender, myrrh, peppermint, pine, rosemary, tea tree
Tonic:	(invigorates)	basil, bergamot, black pepper, cardamom, carrot, clary sage, fennel, frankincense, garlic, geranium, ginger, grapefruit, hyssop, jasmine, juniper, lemon, lemongrass, lime,

mandarin, marjoram, melissa, myrrh, nutmeg, neroli, orange, origanum, parsley, patchouli, pimento, pine, rose, rosemary, sage, sandalwood, tangerine, thyme, verbena, vetivert, yarrow

Uterine: (tonic for the uterus) clary sage, clove, frankincense, jasmine, melissa, myrrh, rose

Vascoconstrictor: (causes contraction of blood vessel walls) cypress, geranium, peppermint

Vasodilator: (causes dilation of blood vessel walls) garlic

Vermifuge: (causes expulsion of worms) basil, bergamot, cajuput, camphor, caraway, carrot, camomile, cinnamon, clove, eucalyptus, fennel, garlic, hyssop, lemon, niaouli, peppermint, tarragon, thyme

Vulnerary: (aids healing of wounds/prevents tissue degeneration) benzoin, bergamot, camphor, camomile, elemi, eucalyptus, frankincense, galbanum, geranium, hyssop, juniper, lavender, marjoram, myrrh, niaouli, origanum, rosemary, tarragon

USEFUL INFORMATION

INFORMATION CENTRES

AOC

International Federation of Aromatherapy (IFA)
Stamford House
2/4 Chiswick High Road
London W4 1TH
TEL: 0181 742 2605

Aromatherapy Organizations Council
3 Latymer Close
Braybrooke
Market Harborough
Leicester LE16 8LN
TEL/FAX: 01858 434242

AROMATHERAPY ASSOCIATIONS

Association of Holistic Therapists
39 Prestbury Road
Cheltenham
Gloucestershire GL25 2PT
TEL: 01242 512601

Association of Medical Aromatherapists
Abergare, Rhu Point
Helensburgh G84 8NF
TEL: 0141 332 4924

Association of Natural Medicine
27 Bruiaintree Road
Witham
Essex CM8 2DD
TEL/FAX: 01376 502 762

Association of Physical and Natural Therapists
68A The Avenue Worcester Park
Surrey KT4 7HJ
TEL: 0181 335 3202

English Société de l'Institut Pierre Franchome, France
Belmont House
Newport
Essex CB11 3RF
TEL: 01799 540622

Holistic Aromatherapy Foundation
83 Harestone Hill
Caterham
Surrey CR3 6DL
TEL: 01883 343419

*International Federation of
   Aromatherapists*
Stamford House
2/4 Chiswick High Road
London W4 1TH
TEL: 0181 742 2605

*International Society of Professional
   Aromatherapists*
Hinckley and District Hospital
Tyhe Annex
Mount Road, Hinckley
Leicestershire LE10 1AG
TEL:01455 890956
FAX: 01455 890956

*Register of Qualified
   Aromatherapists*
23 Castle Street
Tiverton
Devon EX16 6RE
TEL: 01884 243172

*The Academy of Aromatherapy and
   Massage*
50 Cow Wynd
Falkirk
Sterlingshire FK11PU
TEL: 01324 612 658

Micheline Arcier Aromatherapy
7 William Street
London SW1X 9HL
TEL: 0171 235 3545

*Beaumont College of Natural
   Medicine*
16 Dittons Road
Eastbourne
East Sussex BN21 1DW
TEL: 01323 724855

Berkshire School of Natural Therapy
Conifers, 21 Dukes Wood
Crowthrone
Berkshire RG11 6NF
TEL: 01344 761715

The Chalice Foundation
Chalice House
11 Howell Road
Exeter
Devon
EX4 4LG
TEL/FAX: 01392 495050

Sandra Day School of Health Related
  Studies
4 Healey Hall Mews
Shawclough Road
Rochdale
Lancashire OL12 2GG
TEL: 01706 3563328

European College of Natural Medical
  Therapies
16 North Parade
Belfast BT7 2GG
TEL: 01232 641454

Good Scents School of Natural
  Therapies
9 Chute Way
Salvington
Worthing
West Sussex BN13 3EA
TEL: 01903 694202

The School of Holistic Aromatherapy
108B Haverstock Hill
London NW3 2BD
TEL: 0171 284 1315

The Humberside College of
  Aromatherapy
56 Whitstone Close
Bransholme
Hull HU7 4DY
TEL: 01482 835358

Hygeia School of Holistic Therapy
7–9 Springfield Road
Altrincham
Cheshire WA14 1HE
TEL: 0161 941 5027
FAX: 0161 926 8423

The Institute of Traditional Herbal
  Medicine and Aromatherapy
15 Coolhurst Rd (ap 5)
London N8 8EP
TEL: 0181 348 3755

The International Academy of
  Holistic Studies
The Lunny and Worword
  Aromatherapy Program
PO Box 210
Romford
Essex RM7 7DW
TEl/FAX: 01438 357357

Naturecare
16 Sunnyhill Rd,
Streatham
London SW16 2UH
TEL: 0181 664 6150

Shirley Price College of
   Aromatherapy
Headquarters: Essential House
Upper Bond Street
Hinckley
Leicestershire
LE10 IRS
TEL: 01455 615466
FAX: 01455 615054

Purple Flame School of
   Aromatherapy
61 Clinton Lane
Kenilworth
Warwick CV8 !AS
TEL: 01926 55980
FAX: 01926 512001

The Raworth Centre
20–26 South Street
Dorking
Surrey RH4 2HQ
TEL: 01306 742150
FAX: 01306 742163

Renhardou Beauty and Alternative
   Therapy Training Centre
Acorn House
Cherry Orchard House
Croyden
Surrey
TEL: 0181 686 4781
FAX: 0181 649 9291

The Scottish College of
   Complimentary Medicine
11 Park Circus
Glasgow G3 6AX
TEL: 01436 821571

The Tisserand Institute
65 Church Road
Hove
East Sussex BN3 2BD
TEL: 01273 206640
FAX: 01273 329811

There are many other affiliated
training organizations too numer-
ous to include here but for further
details contact the AOC.

SUPPLIERS (BY MAIL):

for essential oils, carrier oils

NEW SEASONS
9 Home Farm
Ardington
Wantage
Oxfordshire OX12 8PN
TEL: 01235 821110
FAX: 01235 834294

FLEUR
Pembroke Studios
Pembroke Road
London
N10 2JE
TEL: 0181 444 7424
FAX: 0181 444 0704

The Tisserand Institute
65 Church Road
Hove
East Sussex
BN3 2BD
TEL: 0273 206640
FAX: 01273 329811

Norman and Germaine Rich
2 Coval Gdns
London SW14 7DG
TEL: 0181 878 2976

FOR MASSAGE COUCHES:

New Concept, Dept AT
Cox Hal Lane
Tattingstone
Ipswich
Suffolk
IP9 2NS
TEL: 01473 328006

The Churchill Centre
22 Montagu Street
London W1H 1TB
TEL: 0171 402 9475

MAGAZINES

The Aromatherapy Quarterly
DEPT.AT
Ranelagh Ave
London
SW13 OBY

Aromatherapy Times
IFA office
2–4 Chiswick High Road
London
W4 1TH

Aromatherapy World
Hinckley and District Hospital and Health Centre
The Annexe
Mount Road
Hinckley
Leics LE10 IAG
TEL: 01455 637987
FAX: 01455 890956

VIDEOS

Valerie Worwood:
Essentially Yours
PO Box 38 Romford
RM1 DN

Shirley Price's Aromatherapy and Massage
Distributed by M.C.E.G/Virgin Vision Limited

PRINCIPLES OF TAROT

EVELYNE AND TERRY DONALDSON

Tarot has fascinated people for hundreds of years, but at times the symbolism can be difficult to relate to our contemporary lives. This introductory guide demystifies the tarot and clearly explains:

- the meaning of each card

- how to do a reading for yourself and other people

- how to use the tarot as a tool for personal development

- easy ways of gaining a deeper understanding of this ancient art

Evelyne and Terry Donaldson are highly experienced tarot teachers and readers. They run the London Tarot Training Centre. Terry Donaldson is the author of *Step by Step Tarot*, also published by Thorsons, co-creator of the Dragon Tarot deck and Wyvern, the game of Dragons, Dragon-Slayers and Treasure.

PRINCIPLES OF NLP

JOSEPH O'CONNOR AND IAN MCDERMOTT

Neuro-Linguistic Programming (NLP) is the psychology of excellence. It is based on the practical skills that are used by all good communicators to obtain excellent results. These skills are invaluable for personal and professional development. This introductory guide explains:

- what NLP is

- how to use it in your life personally, spiritually and professionally

- how to understand body language

- how to achieve excellence in everything that you do

Joseph O'Connor is a trainer, consultant and software designer. He is the author of the bestselling *Introducing NLP* and several other titles, including *Successful Selling with NLP* and *Training with NLP*.

Ian McDermott is a certified trainer with the Society of Neuro-Linguistic Programming. He is the Director of Training for International Teaching Seminars, the leading NLP training organization in the UK.

PRINCIPLES OF
THE ENNEAGRAM

KAREN WEBB

There is a growing fascination with the Enneagram – the ancient uncannily accurate model of personality types linking personality to spirit. Most people can recognize themselves as one of the nine archetypes. This introduction to the subject explains:

- the characteristics of the nine types

- how the system works

- ways of understanding your own personality

- how to discover your true potential and attain it

- ways to enhance your relationships

Karen Webb is an experienced Enneagram teacher, counsellor and workshop leader. She has introduced many people to the system and guided them in using the information to change their lives. She has been employed by many large companies as a management consultant.

PRINCIPLES OF
HYPNOTHERAPY

VERA PEIFFER

Interest in hypnotherapy has grown rapidly over the last few years. Many people are realizing that it is an effective way to solve problems such as mental and emotional trauma, anxiety, depression, phobias and confidence problems, and eliminate unwanted habits such as smoking. This introductory guide explains:

- what hypnotherapy is

- how it works

- what its origins are

- what to expect when you go for treatment

- how to find a reputable hypnotherapist

Vera Peiffer is a leading authority on hypnotherapy. She is a psychologist in private practice in West London specializing in analytical hypnotherapy and a member of the Corporation of Advanced Hypnotherapy.

PRINCIPLES OF PAGANISM

VIVIANNE CROWLEY

Interest in Paganism is steadily increasing and, while rooted in ancient tradition, it is a living religious movement. With its reverence for all creation, it reflects our current concern for the planet. This introductory guide explains:

- what Paganism is

- the different Pagan paths

- what Pagans do

- how to live as a Pagan

Vivianne Crowley is the author of the bestselling *Wicca: The Old Religion in the New Millennium*. She is a priestess, a teacher of the Pagan way and a leading figure in western Paganism. She has a doctorate in psychology and has trained in transpersonal therapy.

PRINCIPLES OF
NUTRITIONAL THERAPY

Environmental pollutants and the use of antibiotics and other drugs cause changes in the body which can affect its ability to absorb and assimilate nutrients. Widespread nutritional deficiencies causing much chronic illness have resulted from this in our society. Nutritional therapists, complementary medicine practitioners working with special dies and vitamins, are often able to cure illnesses such a eczema, chronic fatigue, premenstrual syndrome, irritable bowel syndrome, hyperactivity and migraine.

This introductory guide explains:

- how deficiencies occur

- how nutritional therapy works

- which key illnesses the therapy can fight

Linda Lazarides is Director of the Society for the Promotion of Nutritional Therapy. She is a practising nutritional therapist with several years of working with a GP. She is an advisor to the Institute of Complementary Medicine and BACUP and is on the advisory panel of *Here's Health* magazine.

PRINCIPLES OF
SELF-HEALING

DAVID LAWSON

In these high pressure times we are in need of ways of relaxing and gaining a sense of happiness and peace. There are many skills and techniques that we can master to bring healing and well-being to our minds and bodies.

This introductory guide includes:

- visualizations to encourage our natural healing process

- affirmations to guide and inspire

- ways of developing the latent power of the mind

- techniques for gaining a deeper understanding of yourself and others

David Lawson is a teacher, healer and writer. He has worked extensively with Louise Hay, author of *You Can Heal Your Life*, and runs workshops throughout the world. He is the author of several books on the subject, including *I See Myself in Perfect Health*, also published by Thorsons.

PRINCIPLES OF TAROT	0 7225 3217 2	£5.99
PRINCIPLES OF NLP	0 7225 3195 8	£5.99
PRINCIPLES OF THE ENNEAGRAM	0 7225 3191 5	£5.99
PRINCIPLES OF HYPNOTHERAPY	0 7225 3242 3	£5.99
PRINCIPLES OF PAGANISM	1 85538 507 4	£5.99
PRINCIPLES OF NUTRITIONAL THERAPY	0 7225 3285 7	£5.99
PRINCIPLES OF SELF-HEALING	1 85538 486 8	£5.99

All these books are available from your local bookseller or can be ordered direct from the publishers.

To order direct just tick the titles you want and fill in the form below:

Name: _____

Address: _____

_____

Postcode: _____

Send to Thorsons Mail Order, Dept 3, HarperCollinsPublishers, Westerhill Road, Bishopbriggs, Glasgow G64 2QT.

Please enclose a cheque or postal order or your authority to debit your Visa/Access account —

Credit card no: _____

Expiry date: _____

Signature: _____

— up to the value of the cover price plus:
UK & BFPO: Add £1.00 for the first book and 25p for each additional book ordered.

Overseas orders including Eire: Please add £2.95 service charge. Books will be sent by surface mail but quotes for airmail dispatches will be given on request.

24–HOUR TELEPHONE ORDERING SERVICE FOR ACCESS/VISA CARD-HOLDERS — TEL: 0141 772 2281.